Lead, Drive, and Thrive in the System

2nd Edition

by Jennifer S. Mensik Kennedy, PhD, MBA, RN, NEA-BC, FAAN

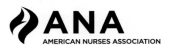

American Nurses Association
Silver Spring, Maryland • 2023

ANA
AMERICAN NURSES ASSOCIATION

Lead, Drive, and Thrive in the System, 2nd Edition.
The American Nurses Association (ANA) is the premier national professional association representing the interests of the nurses of the United States. ANA is the only full-service professional organization representing the interests of the nation's 4.2 million registered nurses through its constituent member nurses associations and its organizational affiliates. ANA advances the nursing profession by fostering high standards of nursing practice, promoting a safe and ethical work environment, bolstering the health and wellness of nurses, and advocating on health care issues that affect nurses and the public. ANA is at the forefront of improving the quality of health care for all.

American Nurses Association
8515 Georgia Avenue, Suite 400
Silver Spring, MD 20910-3492
1-800-274-4ANA
http://www.nursingworld.org

Library of Congress Control Number: 2023944868

Print: 978-1-953985-04-0
ePDF: 978-1-953985-05-7
ePUB: 978-1-953985-06-4
Mobi: 978-1-953985-08-8

Contents

Chapter 4. Innovation and Standardization

Chapter 8. Systems Thinking from the Corporate Office

Introduction to Systems Thinking and Systems-Based Leadership

"Build a system that even a fool can use, and
only a fool will want to use it."

—George Bernard Shaw

As I update this book 10 years later, the statement, "The more things change the more things stay the same," rings true for the US health care system. The health care industry is making some progressive changes, but we still talk about the future, using the same examples we discussed 10, 20, and 30 years ago about what the future should be. We are slow and hesitant to make many needed changes in our system. For instance, value-based care and bundling payments are not a new concept, but we still talk about them as if they are a new idea or the future.

Health care systems are complex entities created by people. We have all heard our colleagues and maybe even ourselves complain about "the system." Yet, the system is not independent of us; it did not create itself and cannot change by itself. We all co-created the system actively or passively. So, if we actually want a better system, then we are the answer.

There is comfort in the system staying the same and not changing as change is hard and unknown. Real change in the system will impact where clinicians practice, where the money is spent, and how much people are paid. And it will change how and where people will get health care. Change will affect things for everyone, and it will be a trade-off of some better and some worse.

As we do make change happen, it is important to know that no system is ever perfect, and it requires constant interaction, inputs, changes, and adjustments to continue to function at the desired level. Understandably, there are many times when the system fails. However, it should not be the default to just blame the system when something doesn't go right. Each one of us, regardless of our position, has helped create the system we work in, either actively or passively, and is part of the system. This includes knowing a problem exists but not attempting to change or fix the problem.

When I was in my PhD program, I completed a concept analysis. All these years later, I still enjoy thinking about the concept of unintended consequences. This concept—which can be viewed as a law in some instances—is defined in many fields, from economics to other social sciences. *Unintended consequence*, based on the social science usage and sometimes referred to as an *unanticipated consequence* (Merton, 1936), is an outcome that is not actively or purposely intended.

Robert K. Merton, an influential sociologist who first popularized the term, wrote that unintended consequences are caused by any one of these five things (Merton, 1936, pp. 901–903):

1. Ignorance: Lack of knowledge, expertise, experience, and/or prudence

2. Error: Incorrect reasoning or analysis and interpretation of the actual issue

3. Immediacy of interests: Focus on short-term goals only

4. Basic values: Sticking to out-of-date policies or beliefs

5. Self-defeating prophecy: Fear, assuming failure before starting

These potential antecedents are driven in part by the inherent complexity of the systems in which we work. One person or a team cannot possibly know everything

DEFINITIONS	
Culture of safety is where the culture of an organization focuses on the safety of patient care. The culture is such that everyone recognizes and is involved in ensuring safe patient care.	*Just culture* is when someone is not blamed for system failures that they had no individual control over.

we need to know to make a perfect decision; thus, the decisions we all make are based on a principle known as bounded rationality.

Coined by the prolific and pioneering social scientist Herbert A. Simon, bounded rationality is one of several key explanations about decision-making. The rationality of individuals is limited by the information they have, the cognitive limitations of their minds, and the finite amount of time they have to make a decision (Simon, 1957). Due to this bounded ability to make decisions, even the smallest of decisions can have far-reaching intended or unintended effects. Thus, we must always be working on fixing the system.

It is important to note that unintended consequences are not always bad. They could be positive. The bad thing about positive unintended consequences is that you might not be able to replicate them. And in a system, you want to replicate good outcomes! How many times have you witnessed a great outcome or great trending on several data points and no one can explain why?

THINGS TO CONSIDER

To decrease the negative effects of bounded rationality, look at your team structure. This is where interdisciplinary teams can shine! When setting up a team to work on a project, consider who you invite. Think about the system and invite others who are impacted by the work.

1. Do they represent diverse areas of the organization, such as regulatory, security, legal, housekeeping, and finance (just to name a few!)?

2. Does everyone on the team think like you? (Hint: If everyone thinks like you, that will be a problem!)

3. Is there representation on the team from the ones for whom you are trying to solve the issue? (If you are solving a problem for a direct care nurse, they need to be a part of that team.)

THINGS TO CONSIDER

One way to decrease negative effects of unintended consequences is to conduct a premortem. You may have heard about postmortems. A postmortem is a process to identify what did and didn't work after a project is launched while incorporating the lessons learned within the organization. A premortem is a strategy where the team imagines the project or the team itself failed before the launch (during the development stage) and works backward to identify what the causes could be so that in the development of the project, those causes are addressed before the launch.

Unintended consequences and bounded rationality are important concepts to understand as you go into this book. Together, these terms reconfirm that no one knows everything, that all of us make decisions that are bounded by incomplete knowledge or time, and that any of our decisions (or lack thereof) could have unintended consequences. It also demonstrates that we need to include others in gathering information and the decision-making process.

As we educate ourselves more about the system and decentralize decision-making, we help create a system that allows everyone the ability to lead from within a system context. So, before you decide to blame the system for anything, reflect on your role in the system. Are you a passive or an active participant within the system? Remember unintended consequences and bounded rationality can go a long way in creating havoc—or greatness!

Before I discuss what this book is about, it is important to clarify what this book is not about. It is not an in-depth book on health policy and economics. But you will see throughout this book how they interact and influence the health system. You will be able to see how health policy may influence an organization or the nurse as it trickles down in the system! There are many settings for and types of organizations that provide health care services. This book is not strictly about hospitals or hospital systems, and you will read tips and considerations that traverse the continuum of the health care system.

About This Book

This book covers a wide range of topics and issues that are important to all nurses. We are all a part of the system. Some of the material covered is relevant to single organizations, units, teams, managers, executives, and staff not employed in a system. However, all the information builds to understanding how to lead within any system, including academia, health providers, nonprofit organizations, and others. This book is not intended to cover everything one might need to know to lead, drive, and thrive in the system, but it is a good start!

- *Chapter 1:* "Introduction to Health Care Systems" introduces health care systems, collaboration, change, and why a system needs to work together. By the end of the chapter, I hope you will start to see things a little differently than when you started this book!

- *Chapter 2:* "Our Evolving Health Care System" discusses our ever-changing world related to health care reform; accountable care; the care continuum; and federal, local, private, public, regulatory, and accreditation organizations that influence the health care systems we work in.

- *Chapter 3:* "What Is Systems Thinking?" is definitely more scientific and theory based in nature. Do not worry: I do not want to lose anyone in this chapter. My goal is to discuss systems thinking, science, and theory in a manner in which you can understand and use in your own understanding of the world.

- *Chapter 4:* "Innovation and Standardization" discusses what innovation is, what standardization is, and how and why you need to bring the two together!

- *Chapter 5:* "Facilitating and Managing Change" is about change, components to consider, and how to facilitate change so that we are successful.

- *Chapter 6:* "All Nurses Are Leaders" discusses the nurse as a leader and breaks down nurse leadership by roles. Read each section to understand what others might be going through in their leadership roles and what others have learned, and take from it what you can to continue your growth as a leader.

- *Chapter 7:* "Systems Thinking from an Individual Organization Up" focuses on the individual in a department or single organization working their way up and between levels, departments, or organizations.

- *Chapter 8:* "Systems Thinking from the Corporate Office Down" discusses the role of the corporate or system employee in the health care system. We will also discuss the issues with top-down and bottom-up approaches in decision-making and how to navigate these potential issues in addition to system-level team development.

- *Chapter 9:* "Moving Everyone Forward" will focus on how to move the whole organization forward through strategic thinking, planning, and being one.

Throughout the book, you will read about theory and practice, build a deeper understanding of the open systems in which we all work, and hear stories from nurses and individuals who have gained their own insights and experienced "ah ha" moments about what it means to work in a system.

CHAPTER 1

Introduction to Health Care Systems

"Everything must be made as simple as possible.
But not simpler."

—Albert Einstein

Welcome to *Lead, Drive, and Thrive in the System*, a book about how nurses can lead from any position or level in the system. Leading, driving, and thriving in any system is a very operational, tactical, and thoughtful process. Throughout this book, I will refer to the "system," by which I mean any system involved, directly or indirectly, in health care. This could include (but is not limited to) an individual department or facility, academia, government, health insurers, e-commerce, and large multistate horizontally or vertically integrated organizations.

The integration could consist of only hospitals, only clinics, only home care agencies, only nursing homes, only pharmacies, and so on, as well as any combination of all the above. Everything and everyone is connected and part of a system.

Chapter 1 will introduce health care systems, collaboration, change, and why a system needs all its members to work together. By the end of the chapter, I hope you will start to see things a little differently than when you started this book! Many concepts in this chapter will be expounded later in this book.

What Is Leading, Driving, and Thriving in the System?

All nurses are leaders regardless of role, position, or educational level. A clinical, direct-care RN leads by providing care as part of the interdisciplinary team, most importantly through the professional role of care coordinator and patient advocate. Additionally, the nurse delegates tasks to others on the care team and may take part in shared leadership. Through those activities, the clinical RN is leading in the part of the system where that RN has responsibility and accountability.

The nurse manager is also a leader. It is not the formal management tasks that make them a leader but their ability to lead change at both higher and lower levels in the system. Regardless of your role as a nurse, all RNs and advanced practice RNs (APRNs) have a professional responsibility to lead.

The responsibility to lead is founded in the American Nurses Association (ANA) *Code of Ethics for Nurses*, which states, "The nurse's primary commitment is the patient, whether an individual, family, group, community, or population" (ANA, 2015). Nurses can have many commitments or loyalties beyond their patient, including loyalty to their employer. This can and does create conflicts for nurses. However, it is important to remember that the nurse–patient relationship is the primary commitment, which supersedes the nurse–employer relationship. This is

---

A CONSIDERATION FOR SYSTEMS THINKING

In my faculty role, one of my favorite system assignments was to have each student use a mind-mapping software to demonstrate the connections between a local individual-level health quality outcome and the clinician, unit, facility, city/county, state, national, and global-level influences. Regardless of where you are, we are truly a system of systems.

A CONSIDERATION FOR SYSTEMS THINKING

Leadership versus Management

Leadership and management are not the same concept and can actually be mutually exclusive. A leader is not necessarily a manager, and a manager is not necessarily a leader.

"In this chaotic world, we need leaders. But we don't need bosses. We need leaders to help us develop the clear identity that lights the dark moments of confusion" (Wheatley, 2006, p. 131).

one of many reasons why the public has voted through the Gallop Poll that nursing is the most trusted profession for over the past 20 years.

The *Code of Ethics for Nurses* does not say "the staff nurse's primary commitment," but "the nurses." This means that regardless of your role, manager, executive, APRN, or staff nurse, your primary commitment is the patient. As a member of the profession and as a nurse, your primary commitment is the patient, regardless of the role you hold, which is the reason the system even exists. If you have a role in nursing as a nurse manager, director, or CNO/CNE, you are automatically given additional responsibilities as you lead in the system; however, the patient is still your primary commitment.

There will be further discussion about different RN and APRN roles related to leading in the system in chapter 6.

Definition of Nursing

This book can be used by nurses and those in other health care disciplines as well. That being said, this book focuses on the role of the professional nurse, so it is appropriate to ensure a standard definition of nursing before continuing. In this book, we will use the ANA definition of nursing.

As per the ANA's Scope and Standards of Nursing Practice (2021), nursing is defined as follows:

> Nursing integrates the art and science of caring and focuses on the protection, promotion, and optimization of health and human functioning; prevention of illness and injury; facilitation of healing; and alleviation of suffering through compassionate presence. Nursing is the diagnosis and treatment of human responses and advocacy in the care of individuals, families, groups, communities, and populations in recognition of the connection of all humanity. (p. 1)

Maybe your organization has its own definition of nursing. We will discuss later in chapter 2 the importance of standardization, but for now, the importance of using a standard definition of nursing is so that all nurses can communicate clearly as one nursing voice. There is an important premise in standardization, and clearly many issues exist in our current health care system due to our reluctance to standardize and desire to personalize things.

To underscore the importance of evidence-based standardization, I will borrow a phrase Lucian Leape, MD, used at a quality conference in 2014: *Autonomy Nuts.*

As a former health policy analysis and professor, he stated that autonomy nuts are people who are familiar with the standards and evidence but choose to ignore them in favor of their own way of doing things. There is a time and place for autonomy, as this concept is vital to the role of the professional RN, but there is also a time and place to support standardized definitions, language, and processes! Standardization can improve our ability to communicate more effectively the outcomes of our work, as it allows us all to work from the same page. Effective communication is vital when you are leading in the system.

A First Look at Systems

Typically, when people think of a health care system, words such as "bureaucratic," "hierarchical," "complex," and "slow" often come to mind.

All of these can be true but it does not mean it has to stifle innovation. And while we may not like hierarchy, complexity, and bureaucracy, they can and do serve a purpose. I believe that the connotation of these words tends to be negative, mostly because people do not know how to navigate and negotiate effectively or have the patience needed to see change through to the end. Once we hit the first barrier, we attach negative feelings to the system. To lead in a system, any system, nurses must know the ins and outs of an organization, the internal and external inputs that influence and mold it, and that anyone can make a difference for change. It is through the bureaucracy and partnering with others that we understand how to most effectively impact the complexity and interrelatedness of the system.

Systems are defined in more detail in chapter 3. However, as an introduction, there are a few ways to think about systems. You should think of systems not only

DEFINITIONS FOR SYSTEMS THINKING

I use the word "practice" throughout the book when referring to work. I find it to be a professional view of nursing as opposed to calling it work, which implies a task-based job. Saying that someone "practices" is not limited to direct-care RNs or APRNs. Educators, leaders, case managers, researchers, and other RNs also have a "practice." For example, an educator practices education and a nurse leader practices leadership. So when I say "practice" anywhere in the book, think about your "work" or "job" through the lens of a professional. I encourage you to use the word "practice" from now on instead of saying "job" or "work." It may feel odd at first, but words are powerful and words change cultures.

as a set of levels but also as a worldview, or a mental model of the world and reality. Systems can also be open or closed. Open systems interact with the world around it, whereas closed do not. Health care is an open system.

When it comes to thinking about levels in a system, James Miller (1978) stated that systems exist at eight "nested" hierarchical levels, which include the cell, organ, organism, group, organization, community, society, and supranational system. Each level works within and between other levels and has its own perspective and specific role to accomplish, neither of which is necessarily better than the other. In this book, we focus on the latter six levels: organism (person), group, organization, community, society (national), and supranational system (global).

Each for their own!

In any organization, individuals at any level may think they have it the hardest or that they need to "fight for their resources." That somehow, their shift/team/unit/ department is not being given the resources needed on purpose. This belief, which is due in part to the culture and management practices of an organization, can lead to the belief that everyone needs to fend for themselves.

While our health care system does continue to grow in costs, it may not feel like additional money or resources are making it downstream or to the lowest level. However, asking for more is not always the best way to achieve what is needed. Is there a way to rearrange what we already use differently, more effectively?

As socially responsible nurses, we cannot afford to let the US health care system continuously increase spending unchecked. We all need to be a part of rethinking how to spend the money that is already spent in health care! Why? Statista (2022) states that 19.7 percent of our gross domestic product (GDP) in the United States was spent on health care in 2020, with the highest spending among developed countries. GDP is an important measure within the US and across countries when it comes to comparing expenditures. GDP is the total monetary value of all goods and services produced in a country at a given time. This is not government spending or tax dollars alone.

DEFINITIONS FOR SYSTEMS THINKING	
System: "A set of components that work together for the overall objective of the whole" (Haines, 1998, p. VI)	*Real Organization:* "A dense network of interdependent relationships" (Wheatley, 2006, p. 144)

For comparison of US health care spending against other areas, for instance, the US budget for the Department of Defense amounted to 3.3 percent of GDP in 2021 (US Congressional Budget Office, 2022) and 3.1 percent of GDP for elementary and secondary public schools' expenditures in 2018 (National Science Foundation [NSF], 2021). US health care spending is estimated to continue to grow to 24.8 percent by 2050 (IHME, 2020). So, the takeaway is the more we spend in one area, the less we must spend in another (or go into debt).

Therein lies the dilemma. If we spend more in health care, what and where do we spend less? And, if we spend more, how much and where? Who gets it? What area or industry is it taken from? Our health care system is an integral part of the lives of everyone in the US. Spending more requires trade-offs. How do we improve our health care system when we already spend more per capita than any other country? All good questions. We need to rethink our system at each level. As we make changes in our health care system, whether in our unit or department, organization, or national policy, we all need to change our own perspectives and take into consideration all other perspectives.

Belonging to a System

While the system may now seem even more daunting, there are numerous benefits to being part of a system. Depending on where you practice, whether at a higher level such as the corporate office (table 1.1) or lower level such as a department in an organization (table 1.2), these issues will vary. The often-quoted idiom "Can't see the forest for the trees," as well as the opposite, "Can't see the trees for the forest," is a good metaphor to understand the positive and negative aspects of being within varying levels of a system. Anyone can fall victim to losing the larger picture, or the details, within a situation.

Change: It Starts with You

How can one change their perspective from *everyone for themselves* to *everyone for our patients and communities*? I know someone is saying, "I fight for myself so that I can give the patients what they deserve!" Fair. But, if we are going to lead change so that we can deliver on the quintuple aim of improving health, improving care experience, reducing the cost of care, advancing health equity, and attaining joy at work (Nundy et al., 2022), we need to think about the system and everyone.

If we are going to lead change so that we can deliver care better in the future as our health care system changes, how can you think differently so that you can still

Table 1.1. Benefits and Potential Issues Practicing at the Corporate Level

BENEFITS	POTENTIAL ISSUES
Stay focused on larger issue	Lose sight of local issues and details
Become and visualize the interconnection across multiple organizations	Have more superficial relationships in lieu of local personal ones
Understand and see strategic plans and visions with greater clarity	Lose sight of how higher-level planning may negatively affect lower levels

Table 1.2. Benefits and Potential Issues Practicing at the Department Level

BENEFITS	POTENTIAL ISSUES
See how end results impact patients and staff directly	Perceived lack of power to make changes that may positively affect staff and patients
Able to visualize and change details	May not understand how localized slight changes could negatively impact policies
Have closer relationships with individuals at closest point of care to patient	May not see the aggregated impact of decisions

advocate and provide for your patients while working as a team? We are all responsible for decreasing the cost of health care in the US.

One way to change your perspective is to start with trust. Trust first that everyone you work with is there for the good of the patient and that everyone's goal is the same. They just may have a different way of getting there. We all have had a different journey and experiences that have given us different perspectives. It is not bad or good, simply different. We all look at situations and events and interpret what other people say and do, comparing it to our own set of past experiences, our culture, faith, values, and so on. These things all helped us to form our beliefs about ourselves, about others, and about the world in which we live. The meaning we give events, the way we make sense of our world, is based upon our set of core beliefs. This set of core beliefs is different for each person. So, seek to understand differences first and build trust upon that!

Sister Facilities

I have worked in multiple health care systems. One of the best lessons I took away from them was how you referred to or "saw" the other organizations in your system.

Often, I would hear people refer to other hospitals, clinics, or home care agencies that were part of "them" in a very negative, patronizing manner—preferring to call their organization the flagship or another label suggesting that the organization was somehow better than the others. This continues the "us versus them" attitude. I heard things like "We do things best," or "They never meet budget," or worse yet: "I wouldn't take my family members there for care." How does this affect the organization's culture, and what does this say about the person who is making the comment? If you want to have a successful health care system, you cannot have an "us versus them" mentality. We have to be here for the patients and all communities. How do we create and support one another so that our patients and communities are the ones who benefit? One of the better ways of solving this issue is to refer to other entities in your system as family. I and others use the term "sister facilities." We all know that we might have a crazy sister or relative in our family, but we will adamantly defend and support them. Thinking of your system as a family begins the change into a culture of cooperation and togetherness rather than one of abuse.

Holding Companies and Operating Companies

In a health care system, it is important to know which type of business entity you are: holding, operating, or even a combination of the two. This plays out in a whole host of things later in this book, so I will just explain the difference here quickly. The fundamental difference is the structure of management and interactions of each separate entity or organization with the parent company. A holding company or system "holds" an organization, which means that it does not control day-to-day operations or activities and that its interest lies in owning assets or obtaining profits from the company it holds. The held company can do its own thing, as long as it continues to make money for the larger holding company or system. Here, you may find it easier to make change happen faster as each individual facility does not need to work necessarily with other sister facilities to agree on a policy or purchasing the same brand of equipment, for instance.

On the other side is an operating company, a more cohesive system in this case. These companies handle all their own day-to-day operations in addition to the assets and profits. Here, organizations prefer standardizing products, policies, and practice standards across many entities, so change will be much more complex. The theory is that standardization of products and policies leads to cost savings with bulk purchases (i.e., medical supplies, pharmaceuticals).

In a holding company, you may have more competition between each other or see little value in collaborating, whereas in an operating company, you will have more collaboration and a greater value is placed on standardization of operating processes.

Competition versus Collaboration

Regardless of the type of health care system, there is competition. Your sister facilities may try to outdo one another on patient outcomes, for instance, and a little competition could be good for everyone, patients and staff. However, how you structure the incentives can have a profound impact on the outcomes of your own organization. While you may not get a bonus or incentive in your role, it is

---

EXPERIENCE FROM THE FIELD

Collaborating within a Health Care System

I recently taught a class for a diverse group of health care executives on Collaborating for Outstanding Results. We talked about the silos that existed in their hospitals and organizations. Then we talked about how to remove the barriers to create trust and build solid relationships. Silos arise when a leader thinks he or she is better than others and wants more resources devoted to their unit, department, or hospital, rather than looking at what is best for the greater good. Competition for scarce resources pits these leaders against each other. Team members in a silo focus internally rather than seeing the whole organization as part of their team. As competition for resources intensifies, essentials like information may be withheld, causing problems in other departments.

Which is recognized, reinforced, and rewarded by your organizational culture: competition or collaboration? Are you willing to confront high performers who lead silos to indicate that their behavior needs to change?

It takes tremendous effort to break down a silo and build trust and collaboration. One of the most effective ways is for the senior leadership to create one or more goals that require the various teams, disciplines, or facilities to work together. Then the reward structure needs to be changed to reward everyone for achieving the common goal, rather than for working toward their competing individual priorities. Several health care organizations have created a systemwide goal of improved patient satisfaction and said that if the metric is reached, all employees receive a bonus or reward. This means that even those who do not have direct patient care are more inclined to support the caregivers to achieve the desired outcome. This generated success and moved the organization closer to a common vision. How can you create common goals that encourage everyone to work together?

Joanne Schlosser, MBA, SPHR, ACC,
author of *The Big Book of Team Coaching*
Games: Quick, Effective Activities to Energize,
Motivate and Guide Your Team to Success

important to understand how this process may work in your organization. The tricky thing is that this is usually not discussed outside of management levels.

One might be able to obtain the information from the strategic plan and how outcomes are structured as well as goal thresholds. If you are in a system that gives yearly bonuses based on performance measures, how are they given? Is the individual's bonus based on their own individual facility or on department performance, or is your individual bonus based on all of the system entities meeting the goals? How does each of those scenarios play out related to competition and collaboration?

I have worked in systems that gave bonuses in both ways. In the system that gave bonuses based on individual facility performance, the goal for everyone was to focus on their own facility and ensure they meet their goals. You might not really care if the other facilities were not making their goals. You might even pride yourself in thinking or saying you are better than another facility. But is that good for any patient? In the system where you only get your bonus if all facilities meet their goals, the focus is 180 degrees different! If your facility is doing great on patient satisfaction scores and another facility is not, that one facility is placing everyone at risk for losing their bonus. So, guess what? People will want to help each other, share learnings, and offer suggestions. Do they need the ability of a particular staff member? Do they lack resources or a program? People are more likely to try to help and more likely to ask for help from the organizations that are doing well. No one wants to be the organization that brings everyone down.

If the organization is offering bonus/incentives, it is usually considered part of the total compensation of the employee. Here, the base salary may be less, while offering a larger bonus/incentive, for a grand larger total to incentivize the individual to meet the organization's goals. I have also worked in organizations that do not offer or believe in management bonuses or incentives. In this type of organization, the salary is much higher, with the belief that if the money issue is off the table, then everyone will be more focused on meeting the goals together.

Health Care as Cottage Industry

At one end of the spectrum in health care is a small collection of well-functioning health care systems, and on the other end is the traditional cottage industry of solo or small-group practices and facilities. Our current health care system has evolved some from its roots as a cottage industry when health care was practiced and managed at a local level (Mercado, 2020), particularly over the past decade. A cottage industry "is essentially a group of nonintegrated, dedicated artisans who eschew standardization" (Swensen et al., 2010). These solo practices represent "a collection of autonomous professionals providing largely self-defined expert care within organizational, payment, and regulatory environments involving conflicting incentives, goals, and objectives" (Shortell & Schmittdiel, 2004, p. 52). Industry experts thought that after the enactment of Medicare in 1965 and, more recently, the Patient Protection and Affordable Care Act of 2010, cost savings and care improvements would materialize faster, forcing the US health care system away from a cottage industry. Unfortunately, this has not been the case, as evidenced by care that is not adaptive to those with chronic illnesses, unsustainable costs, and failure to deliver basic care (Wasson, 2019).

Although other non–health care industries have transformed themselves using tools such as standardization of value-generating processes, performance measurement, and the transparent reporting of quality, the application of these tools to health care is still controversial. Such fears include the loss of autonomy as providers move to "cookbook medicine." However, appropriate standardization is not a loss of professional autonomy, a misinformed focus on the wrong care, or a loss of individual attention and personal touch in care delivery. The application of improvement tools is not only essential to modernizing care delivery but also the key to preserving the values to which our current system aspires (Swensen et al., 2010). Managed care was supposed to bridge the gap between quality and cost reduction, but that did not transpire (Sinnot et al., 2020). The state and federal government, which is the largest payer of health care, is using its size to pursue value-based payments through organized systems such as accountable care organizations and patient-centered medical homes (Sinnott et al., 2020).

Growing evidence highlights the dangers of continuing to operate as a cottage industry. Fragmentation of care has led to suboptimal performance. The gap between established science and current practice is wide.

The transformation from cottage industry to postindustrial care will be facilitated by combining the following three elements: standardizing care, measuring performance, and transparent reporting (Swensen et al., 2010).

The cottage industry concept does not only apply to physician practices. The multiple small home health agencies in your town, each with a small patient census, may also be engaging in this ideology. Even a large single hospital that is not a part of a system can be thought of as a cottage industry participant. Most other types of business do not function within their industry as a stand-alone, as they may not

Us versus Them

How can you effectively lead in a large health care system? When I started my health care career, I was hired as the organizational development and learning director, part of the administration team to work at a large hospital that had been winning the organization's Best of the Best awards frequently. I was told during the interview process that the senior leadership team considered themselves "mavericks" and that they liked to figure out what needed to be done and do it to achieve corporate and patient goals. The system often lagged behind them or did not really approve of their actions, but they were tolerated because results were achieved. I was part of this "us" getting things done and making a difference.

After two years, I had the opportunity to help open a new state-of-the-art hospital within the same system. When I joined that team, the senior leader made clear that "We may not always agree with what corporate tells us but we do what they say, we toe the line." Hmm, two very different examples of "us versus them," rebellious versus compliant, but I was still a part of the "us" getting things done and making a difference.

Fast forward three years and I am reassigned to the corporate office. Now my focus is on system leadership development, change management, and process improvement. Now I am "them." I changed locations and crossed the line from "us" to "them." Where are my loyalties?

This experience at once enabled me to restructure some key change management efforts by creating cross-functional teams from multiple facilities to problem solve. Whether tackling the challenges of a new performance management system or improving the matrix management reporting structure or the cardiac catheter lab process flow, each team consisted of leaders and front-line staff at various levels coming from large and small hospitals, located in rural and urban areas. Everyone's voice needed to be heard. We thought through the necessary changes and then created a new process for the whole. Occasionally, we also needed to create a process variation, based on the needs of a facility, on size, or on resources. This enabled us to achieve better outcomes and greater consistency and minimized the facilities or departments creating a "workaround" as soon as the process was implemented. Getting people to address a common problem together to achieve a workable solution brought pride and camaraderie. It tore down some of the silos and distrust that existed and generated better solutions.

**Joanne Schlosser, MBA, SPHR, ACC,
President of Rising Stars Leadership Coaching**

survive competition. For instance, there are only a handful of computer companies and computer operating systems (i.e., Microsoft Windows, Apple MacOS, Linux). This is because smaller companies merge with others or are acquired to better position themselves to compete in the marketplace and improve efficiencies. The health care industry, from physicians' offices to hospitals to electronic health record vendors, needs to become more efficient to help reduce the amount of waste in health care as we cannot sustain the current growth.

Common Goal: The Patients

The one thing we all have in common is the patient. It is important to remember that as we lead in the system. We want to lead our health care system to changes that will positively impact our patients, families, and our own lives professionally. Creating a patient-centered health care system will break down silos and bring collaboration to our future systems.

Key Points

- The goals of an Accountable Care Organization (ACO) are to coordinate patient care, provide the right care at the right time, avoid unnecessary duplication of services, and prevent medical errors.

- All nurses are leaders regardless of role, position, or educational level.

- To lead in any system, nurses must know the ins and outs of an organization, the internal and external forces that can mold it, and that anyone can make a difference for change.

- We are all responsible for providing efficient and effective quality care while managing the cost of health care in the United States.

- Align incentives for collaboration, not competition.

- Fragmentation makes it more difficult to transform the industry; we should strive for appropriate standardization.

CHAPTER 2

Our Evolving Health Care System

The trouble with life isn't that there is no answer,
it's that there are so many answers.

—Ruth Benedict, American anthropologist

Everywhere you go in the world, the term *health care system* has a different connotation. In the US, it can refer to our mixed payer system of Medicare, Medicaid, and private payer systems. Elsewhere, it might refer more to a universal health care system. While a national system might be the highest level in our health care system, a health care system can also be a local or regional entity that includes the provision of care, as opposed to the payment of care. I will discuss higher and lower levels of organizations and systems more in chapter 3. In this chapter, we will discuss the US health care system, its components, and the organizations that influence it. In order to lead in the system, all nurses need to understand the external environment that influences internal decisions. Additionally, all nurses need to understand that they have a role in the formation of that external environment and that as leaders, they can form appropriate solutions within their own health care setting in addition to sitting on the boards that make those decisions.

Health Care Reform: The Patient Protection and Accountable Care Act

Outside the Medicare Part D expansion, the Patient Protection and Accountable Care Act (PPACA) has been the largest piece of health care legislation since Medicare was created. A discussion on health care systems, let alone leading in the system, cannot take place without understanding this act. It is often referred to by many as the ACA or "Obamacare."

Over the past decade, members of Congress have attempted to overturn the PPACA over 70 times, and the Supreme Court has dismissed cases against it three times. Over time, the PPACA has gained more support as now 55 percent of the public views the act as favorable up from 46 percent in April 2010 (Kirzinger et al., 2022). To undo all the legislation attached to the PPACA just because someone does not like the individual mandate (which is just one provision out of 89) would be a travesty to our system, our patients, and ourselves as nurses.

Even though the PPACA was passed into law in 2010, many individuals, patients, and health care professionals are still confused about the law. As a nurse, if you do not understand the components of this law, you need to educate yourself so you can speak intelligently about it. News sources such as cable TV and newspapers do not talk about the law in its full extent, partly because they do not really understand health care. Websites provide complete factual information about the 2,000-page law and its 89 components in an easy-to-understand format that any nurse can appreciate. One such website is the Kaiser Family Foundation (https://www.kff.org/health-reform/fact-sheet/summary-of-the-affordable-care-act/), which provides a summary of the act along with other information.

While most of the law has been enacted, there will continue to be changes in our health care system for years to come due to the 89 provisions in the PPACA through innovation and payment reform. Some of these changes include a better focus on translational and patient-centered outcomes and will be discussed later in this chapter.

Goals of a Health Care System

A health care system, also sometimes referred to as a health system, is defined by the Agency for Healthcare Quality and Research (AHRQ) and is expected to evolve over time. However, there are different definitions for both.

The definition of a health system used in AHRQ's Compendium of U.S. Health Systems states it is

> as an organization that includes at least one hospital and at least one group of physicians that provides comprehensive care (including primary and specialty care) who are connected with each other and with the hospital through common ownership or joint management. (AHRQ, 2023a, para 5)

The World Health Organization (WHO) provides a larger perspective of the system, defining it as "the sum total of all the organizations, institutions, and resources whose primary purpose is to improve health. A health system needs staff, funds, information, supplies, transport, communications, and overall guidance and direction. And it needs to provide services that are responsive and financially fair, while treating people decently" (World Health Organization [WHO], 2005).

The WHO (2010) notes several key components of a well-functioning health care system. Regardless of the type of health care system you may think about, any well-functioning health care system responds in a balanced way to a population's needs and expectations by

- Improving the health status of individuals, families, and communities

- Defending the population against what threatens its health

- Protecting people against the financial consequences of ill health

- Providing equitable access to people-centered care

The Continuum of Care

Many health care systems have tended to be hospital centric. We cannot, however, continue to have a "system" that ignores the continuum of care. Our system has to stop being a system of sick care and move to being a system that is not hospital centric but acknowledges and supports the community settings as the primary setting for health care and understands that hospitals are there for when a patient needs more than primary care.

Every generation believes they are living in the most challenging of times, but for health care, we are indeed at a pivotal point. With the health care reform act, legislators are trying to make some type of change. Whatever side you are on, we all agree health care cannot continue down the same path! We need to find innovative ways to provide quality patient care with the money that is already spent on health care in the US. The Centers for Disease Control and Prevention (CDC) notes that in 2019, the US spent $11,582 per capita on health care (CDC/National Center for Health Statistics, 2022). Additionally, of the total spent, 31.4 percent of total expenditures were for hospital care (CDC/National Center for Health Statistics, 2022).

Of our total health care spending, it has been estimated that 25 percent of our spending is on waste (Shrank et al., 2019). Waste is defined as failure of care delivery, failure of care coordination, and administrative complexity as examples (Shrank et al., 2019).

A review (Shrank et al., 2019) computed the following estimated ranges for the cost of waste:

- Failure of care delivery, $102.4 billion to $165.7 billion

- Failure of care coordination, $27.2 billion to $78.2 billion

- Overtreatment or low-value care, $75.7 billion to $101.2 billion

- Pricing failure $230.7 billion to $240.5 billion

- Fraud and abuse, $58.5 billion to $83.9 billion

- Administrative complexity, $265.6 billion

While there has been effort to address waste in numerous studies, no studies through 2019 focused on interventions to decrease administrative complexity (Shrank et al., 2019).

To lead change, hospitals can no longer be considered the primary site of health care in our US health care system. Health care systems that were largely made up of hospitals are now acquiring, merging, or partnering with all settings of health care, recognizing that the only way to be a system and provide accountable care is through a continuum of care. Accountable care organizations (ACOs) made a

---

A CONSIDERATION FOR SYSTEMS THINKING

Practice Terminology and Practice Change

As a home health director, I never understood why people continuously wanted to think of home health care services as "postacute services" only. Why could they not be "preacute services" as well? Change the words you use, and you will change practice!

giant leap forward in making preventative services and primary care a larger piece of the puzzle.

Accountable Care Organizations (ACOs)

Part of this shift in thinking across the continuum and beyond hospitals came from ACOs. The Centers for Medicare & Medicaid Services (CMS) has established a Medicare Shared Savings Program that hopes to facilitate coordination and cooperation among providers to improve the quality of care for Medicare Fee-for-Service (FFS) beneficiaries and reduce unnecessary costs.

This program is known as the Medicare Shared Savings Program (MSSP) with ACOs being a type of program under the MSSP.

To participate in the MSSP, a group of eligible providers, hospitals, and suppliers come together through contracts to form an ACO. The CMS defines ACOs as groups of doctors, hospitals, and other health care providers who come together voluntarily to give coordinated high-quality care to their Medicare patients (CMS, 2022a). The goal of the ACO is to ensure that patients get the right care at the right time, while avoiding unnecessary duplication of services and preventing medical errors (CMS, 2022a). When an ACO succeeds in both delivering high-quality care and spending health care dollars more wisely, the ACO will share in the savings it achieves for the Medicare program (CMS, 2022a). As of 2022, there are 483 Shared Savings Program ACOs providing care to 11 million beneficiaries (CMS, 2022b).

In this program, the ACO agrees to be held accountable for quality, cost, and experience of care for an assigned Medicare FFS beneficiary population. Through financial incentives, the program forces groups to work together as a system for the benefit of the patient and the system.

The Shared Savings Program is designed to improve beneficiary outcomes and increase value of care by

- Promoting accountability for the care of Medicare FFS beneficiaries

- Requiring coordinated care for all services provided under Medicare FFS

- Encouraging investment in infrastructure and redesigned care processes

The Shared Savings Program will reward ACOs that decrease their health care costs while meeting performance standards on quality of care and putting patients first. The CMS definition of an ACO is "an organization of health care providers that agrees to be accountable for the quality, cost, and overall care of Medicare beneficiaries who are enrolled in the traditional fee-for-service program who are assigned to it" (CMS, 2012).

An ACO can include any and all health care–related organizations, including but not limited to clinics, hospitals, insurance payers, home health agencies, dialysis centers, and nursing homes. It makes sense for health care organizations to partner and work together. Why can they not just do this, or why have they not done this before now? The program is designed to allow these partnerships to exist without violating federal laws on trusts and monopolies that govern appropriate competition in the health care marketplace.

The process of becoming a Medicare-acknowledged ACO is responsible for helping to remove legal barriers many organizations face in their transition from cottage to system: the legislation against trusts and monopolies. Prior legislation and regulations allowed some development of clinical service monopolies through certificate-of-need programs, while federal antitrust enforcers have promoted free-market competition that does not allow the health care system to grow or merge like other industries such as phone providers or airline industries.

A CONSIDERATION FOR SYSTEMS THINKING

You may be wondering, what stops more groups from coming together to form these types of systems without participating in the MSSP? The concern is over becoming a monopoly within a service area and violating antitrust laws. Antitrust laws prevent and control the formation of monopolies. Think about the purpose of the board game Monopoly. This is when a company or group has a majority and/or exclusive control over a service or commodity. Often people hear about mergers or acquisitions of hospitals or clinics. The Federal Trade Commission (FTC) reviews these before they are finalized to determine if they would become a

monopoly. If so, then the organization cannot move forward with the merger or acquisition.

What is wrong with monopolies? Monopolies can control and increase prices that consumers pay while decreasing quality, giving consumers little to no alternative. When a proposed ACO submits an application for an MSSP to form an ACO, they can participate in a voluntary expedited antitrust review through the Department of Justice and FTC. However, since it is voluntary, the FTC will continue to monitor aggregated claims data for all ACOs and monitor complaints about ACOs' conduct (FTC, 2011).

If your organization moves toward an ACO model of care, whether obtaining a legally defined status or not, there will be an impact on how you organize and provide care. Becoming an ACO may have these potential impacts for your unit or department regardless of the setting:

- Shorter lengths of stay

- Increased utilization of postacute services

- Increased transparency of your quality measures to other organizations in the ACO

- Shared reimbursement for a patient, potentially meaning less reimbursement for acute care services than received today

- Redesign of care delivery on your unit

In order to be successful in a Shared Saving Program and to reduce health care spending in particular, an ACO, working with the knowledge that acute care hospitalizations take a majority of health care dollars, will need to reduce hospital admissions, not just readmissions. From there, more nursing care will be needed outside of the hospital walls to coordinate care among all these providers, opening more positions outside the hospital walls as well as decreasing the number of nurses needed to provide acute care nursing (Mensik, 2013).

Influential Organizations and Agencies in the US Health Care System

Regardless of the level of the health care system in which you work, there are organizations that do not provide patient care but are influential. This influence may be through regulation, accreditation, professional associations, and policy guidance that are directly or indirectly influential.

The World Health Organization (WHO)

WHO is the directing and coordinating authority for health within the United Nations system. WHO connects nations, partners, and people to promote health, keep the world safe, and serve the vulnerable so that everyone, everywhere can attain the highest level of health (WHO, 2023a). WHO leads efforts to expand universal health care and to coordinate the world's response to health emergencies (WHO, 2023a). A main initiative is the Triple Billion plan, which seeks to improve the future of public health through measurable impacts (WHO, 2023b).

- Target: 1 billion more people better protected from health emergencies

- Target: 1 billion more people enjoying better health and well-being

- Target: 1 billion more people benefiting from universal health coverage

The WHO has a Triple Billion dashboard that can be found at https://portal.who .int/triplebillions/.

National Academy of Medicine (NAM), Formerly the Institute of Medicine (IOM)

The National Academy of Medicine (NAM), formerly the Institute of Medicine (IOM), is an independent, nonprofit organization that works outside of the government to provide unbiased and authoritative advice to decision makers and the public. Established in 1970, NAM is the health arm of the National Academy of Sciences, which was chartered under President Abraham Lincoln in 1863. The mission is to improve health for all by advancing science, accelerating equity, and providing independent, authoritative, and trusted advice nationally and globally (NAM, 2023).

NAM is known for such works as *To Err Is Human: Building a Safer System* (2000 and *Crossing the Quality Chasm: A New Health System for the 21st Century* (2001), as well as the Future of Nursing 2020–2030 report.

Patient-Centered Outcomes Research Institute (PCORI)

The Patient-Centered Outcomes Research Institute (PCORI) is the leading funder of patient-centered comparative clinical effectiveness in the US (PCORI, 2023). Through comparative effectiveness research (CER) funding, PCORI helps people make informed health care decisions and improves health care delivery and outcomes. This is done by ensuring both patients and health care stakeholders participate in the research process through helping prioritize research topics. CERs could include comparing two or more medical treatments, services, or health practices.

Since its authorization by Congress in 2010 as part of the PPACA, PCORI has awarded over $3 billion to nearly 2,000 studies and projects. Results are posted weekly and can be found at https://www.pcori.org/explore-our-portfolio.

Congressional Budget Office

The Congressional Budget Office (CBO) is a nonpartisan agency that produces independent analyses of budgetary and economic issues to support the congressional budget process each year. Each year, the agency produces 600 to 800 cost estimates. A cost estimate states the effects of proposed legislation on the federal budget. These reports inform Congress on what they may ultimately decide to fund.

Even though legislation is passed, it may not actually be funded and moves into a dormant state. An example is the National Health Care Workforce Commission that was established in 2010 under the ACA. As of 2023, it remains dormant, as Congress has never appropriated the $3 million request to fund the commission.

The CBO also has produced numerous reports on a single-payer system. One recent report, *Economic Effects of Five Illustrative Single-Payer Health Care Systems*, found that a single-payer system would decrease administrative waste as well as increase longevity and labor productivity as people's health outcomes improved (Nelson, 2022).

MedPAC and MACPAC

Two other important independent, nonpartisan congressional agencies are the Medicare Payment Advisory Commission (MedPAC) and Medicaid and CHIP Payment and Access Commission (MACPAC). Both agencies produce two reports to Congress yearly that contain recommendations to improve Medicare and Medic-aid/Children's Health Insurance Program (CHIP) programs.

MedPAC was established by the Balanced Budget Act of 1997 to advise the US Congress on issues affecting the Medicare program. In addition to advising on payments, MedPAC provides information on access to care, quality of care, and other issues affecting Medicare. MACPAC advises the Secretary of the US Department of Health and Human Services and the states on a wide array of issues affecting Medicaid and the state CHIP. Both provide an independent source of information, including payment, eligibility, enrollment and retention, coverage, access to care, and quality of care.

Agency for Healthcare Research and Quality (AHRQ)

The Agency for Healthcare Research and Quality (AHRQ) exists within the Department of Health and Human Services. The mission of AHRQ is to "produce evidence to make healthcare safer, higher quality, more accessible, equitable, and affordable, and to work within the U.S. Department of Health and Human Services and with other partners to make sure that the evidence is understood and used" (AHRQ, 2022, para. 1). This is completed through three core competencies: health systems research, practice improvement, and data and analytics (AHRQ, 2019). One major center within this agency is the Evidence-based Practice Center (EPC), which provides reports that may be used for informing and developing coverage decisions, quality measures, educational materials and tools, clinical practice guidelines, and research agendas (AHRQ, 2023b).

National Quality Forum (NQF)

The National Quality Forum (NQF) is a nonprofit, nonpartisan, public service organization that works to catalyze improvements in health care. Specifically, the NQF sets standards, recommends measures for use in payment and public reporting programs, and advances electronic measurement (NQF, 2023a). This is accomplished by ensuring the health care measures that it endorses continue to meet rigorous measurement evaluation criteria. Over 400 organizations from all avenues in health care are members and contribute to this work, including insurance agencies, hospitals, professional associations, trade associations, consumers, health care professionals, and other quality improvement organizations.

While you may not have known about the NQF, you have been impacted by their work. Once a measure is endorsed by the NQF, it can be used by health care systems, health organizations, and government agencies such as the CMS for public reporting and quality improvement activities. Endorsed measures may become required data sets for the CMS. While the CMS is not statutorily required to base decisions related to program use of measures on NQF endorsement status, these measures tend to be generally regarded as a high-quality measure.

NQF-endorsed measures include items such as the following:

- Acute myocardial infarction mortality rate

- 30-day all-cause readmission rate

- Function change: change in mobility score for skilled nursing facilities

- Falls with injury

One can search through all the current NQF-endorsed standards on their website, https://www.qualityforum.org/Measures_List.aspx.

The NQF reviews, endorses, and recommends use of standardized health care performance measures. Performance measures (PMs), which are called *quality measures* by some, are used to evaluate how well health care services are being delivered by comparing different organizations. The NQF's endorsed measures are often invisible to the direct-care RNs, except as additional charting requirements, department-level evidence-based practice projects, or department-level tracking of nurse-sensitive indicators, but these PMs influence the care delivered to millions of patients every day.

The NQF is the only consensus-based health care organization in the nation as defined by the Office of Management and Budget (NQF, 2023b). Nurses and professional associations such as the American Nurses Association not only submit measures for consideration but also sit on these NQF committees that discuss, review, and vote for the adoption of measures.

Nurses who have interest or seek involvement in these areas should follow the development of these measures on the NQF website to provide comments and feedback when solicited.

Institute for Healthcare Improvement (IHI)

The Institute for Healthcare Improvement (IHI) is an independent not-for-profit organization that is known as a driver of results in health and health care improvement worldwide using improvement science (IHI, 2023a). The IHI was officially founderd in 1991, but work began in the late 1980s as part of the National Demonstration Project on Quality Improvement in Health Care focused on redesigning health care into a system without errors, waste, delays, and unsustainable costs (IHI, 2023a).

Over the past 30 years, the IHI has partnered with innovators, leaders, and frontline practitioners around the globe to create bold innovations to improve the health of individuals and populations. To advance their mission, IHI's work is focused in four key areas:

- Pursuing Safe and High-Quality Care

- Improving the Health of Populations

- Building the Capability to Improve

- Innovating and Sparking Action (IHI, 2023a)

The IHI is best known for its innovative development of the Triple Aim. The Triple Aim consists of

- Improving the patient experience of care (including quality and satisfaction)

- Improving the health of populations

- Reducing the per capita cost of health care (IHI, 2023b)

The IHI notes that no one person is accountable for all three dimensions and that all three need to be addressed at the same time to make sustainable change to the US health care system (IHI, 2023b). Since the development of the Triple Aim, additional reiterations have evolved, including the quadruple (including professional wellness) and quintuple (advancing health equity) aims (Nundy et al., 2022).

National Quality Strategy (NQS)

The National Quality Strategy (NQS) was first published in March 2011 as the National Strategy for Quality Improvement in Health Care and is led by the AHRQ on behalf of the US Department of Health and Human Services (DHHS). Developed as a result of the PPACA, the NQS was created through a participatory, transparent, and collaborative process that invited input from a range of stakeholders, including comments from both nurses and the public on a proposed approach to the effort and a draft set of principles and priorities (AHRQ, 2014). As a result, more than 300 groups, organizations, and individuals representing all sectors of the health care industry and the general public provided comments. Based on this input, the NQS established a set of three overarching aims that builds on the IHI's

Triple Aim. These aims will be used to guide and assess local, state, and national efforts to improve health and the quality of health care.

- **Better Care:** Improve the overall quality, by making health care more patient centered, reliable, accessible, and safe.

- **Healthy People/Healthy Communities:** Improve the health of the US population by supporting proven interventions to address behavioral, social, and environmental determinants of health in addition to delivering higher-quality care.

- **Affordable Care:** Reduce the cost of quality health care for individuals, families, employers, and government. (AHRQ, 2014)

Furthermore, to advance these aims, the NQS will focus initially on six priorities:

- Making care safer by reducing harm caused in the delivery of care

- Ensuring that each person and family is engaged as partners in their care

- Promoting effective communication and coordination of care

- Promoting the most effective prevention and treatment practices for the leading causes of mortality, starting with cardiovascular disease

- Working with communities to promote wide use of best practices to enable healthy living

- Making quality care more affordable for individuals, families, employers, and governments by developing and spreading new health care delivery models (AHRQ, 2014)

Centers for Medicare & Medicaid Services (CMS)

The CMS is an agency within the US DHHS responsible for the administration of several key federal health care programs. The CMS, previously known as the Health Care Financing Administration (HCFA), was created in 1977. From 1965 to 1977, the Social Security Administration (SSA) was responsible for administering Medicare. The name was changed from HCFA to CMS in 2001. Marilyn Tavenner, RN, served as the administrator of the CMS from 2011 to 2015.

The CMS hosts the biggest health care programs in the US, Medicare and Medicaid. In addition, the CMS oversees CHIP, the federal and state health insurance marketplaces, the Health Insurance Portability and Accountability Act (HIPAA), and the Clinical Laboratory Improvement Amendments (CLIA), among other services. The CMS is also developing new programs and tools as a result of the PPACA to help organizations and providers deliver better care such as the Medicare Shared Savings Program and ACOs.

Measurement Organizations

Private and public organizations may suggest, and some even determine, quality reporting indicators. As we discuss in later chapters, it is important to consider which data are being collected, from which level, and to ensure appropriate interpretations of the data. Multiple databases of data that your organization may collect are important for you to know and review. Often, we think of data and measurements from an outcome's lens only. However, measures should be thought of in categories of structure, processes, and outcomes based on the Donabedian model (Donabedian, 1988).

- National Patient Safety Goals (Joint Commission)

- National Database for Nursing Quality Indicators (NDNQI)

- CMS Core Measures

- Leapfrog Group

- The Healthcare Effectiveness Data and Information Set (HEDIS)

- Additional state-specific requirements

Regulatory Agencies

Health care is the most regulated of all industries in the US. However, this industry has the closest impact on individuals and their health. What causes the complexity in health care regulations is that they are developed and implemented not only by all levels of government—federal, state, and local—but also by private organizations. In the following section, we will review federal and state regulations and touch on accrediting bodies, which are those private organizations that may add on to the minimum regulations that are really voluntary in nature.

Important laws that regulate health care include the following:

- The federal Health Insurance Portability and Accountability Act of 1996 (HIPAA)

- The Health Information Technology for Economic and Clinical Health (HITECH) Act, enacted in 2009

- The Emergency Medical Treatment and Labor Act (EMTALA), enacted in 1986

- The federal Anti-Kickback Statute (AKBS)

- The Patient Safety and Quality Improvement Act of 2005 (PSQIA)

Federal regulation is one of the basic tools government uses to carry out public policy as well as force innovation. Agencies create regulations (also known as "rules") when Congress provides the authority to do so. The public, which includes health care professionals and organizations, as well as individual citizens, plays an extremely important role in the rulemaking process by commenting on proposed rules. Comments can help shape the decisions and measures used.

Federal Regulations and DHHS Divisions

The DHHS administers 115 programs across its 11 operating divisions and aims to "enhance the health and well-being of all Americans, by providing for effective health and human services and by fostering sound, sustained advances in the sciences underlying medicine, public health, and social services" ("About HHS," 2023).

After congressional bills become laws, federal agencies are responsible for putting those laws into action through regulations or rules. The public has a chance to provide comments on regulations and rules, but you may be wondering how one can keep track of when and where to look for calls for public comments. The *Federal Register* is a daily publication of the US federal government that issues proposed and final administrative regulations of federal agencies. This document provides direction on how to submit comments for proposed regulation. The DHHS receives many comments on proposed rules each year, and all are read. The DHHS has multiple operating divisions that solicit feedback:

- Administration for Children and Families (ACF)

- Administration for Community Living (ACL), formerly the Administration on Aging, ACF's Administration on Developmental Disabilities, and the Office on Disability

- Agency for Healthcare Research and Quality (AHRQ)

- Centers for Disease Control and Prevention (CDC)

- Centers for Medicare & Medicaid Services (CMS)

- Food and Drug Administration (FDA)

- Health Resources and Services Administration (HRSA)

- Indian Health Service (IHS)

- National Institutes of Health (NIH)

- Substance Abuse Mental Health Services Administration (SAMHSA)

Each of these divisions has a website through the HHS.gov site, where you can see all rules as well as the rules open for comment. Here, you can also post your comments on proposed rules and changes. You can even place your name and email on a list to receive updates to those divisions that are most important to you. Remember that with comments open to the public, not every commenter is a nurse and therefore may lack the insights a nurse would have. It is important to voice your opinion, your knowledge, and your views and to help be a part of how we all can shape our health care system.

The DHHS is a very large organization and has many more organizations that report up through it. I find organizational charts helpful in understanding reporting structures, and the federal government is no different (https://www.hhs.gov/about/agencies/orgchart/index.html).

Accreditation Bodies

Many individuals think of The Joint Commission (TJC), Det Norske Veritas (DNV), or Community Health Accreditation Program (CHAP) when the word "regulatory" is mentioned. However, they are actually accreditation bodies. These are important agencies that assist in the regulatory process by surveying the rules on behalf of the CMS. A private organization can have deemed status. Deemed status means that a health care organization met the eligibility requirements for participating in and receiving payment from Medicare or Medicaid programs, including a certification of compliance with the Conditions of Participation (CoPs) or Conditions for Coverage (CfCs) for health care suppliers, which are set forth in federal regulations. The certification is based on a survey conducted by a state agency on behalf of the CMS or by a national accrediting organization, such as TJC, that has been approved by the CMS as having standards and a survey process that meets or exceeds Medicare's CoPs or CfCs and federal survey requirements. Health care organizations that achieve accreditation through a TJC-deemed status survey are determined to meet Medicare and Medicaid requirements. The CMS selects a small, random sample of deemed organizations for visits from accrediting organizations throughout the year. The deemed status is determined within 60 days of the visit to ensure quality.

Personal Pet Peeve Note: Please stop calling The Joint Commission, "JCAHO." They stopped using that name in 2007! While it may be hard to break habits, many younger health care professionals (who graduated after 2007) are learning the wrong name, and it makes the user of old term sound uninformed. That would be like hearing someone still call CMS, "HCFA."

For most types of health care providers or suppliers, accreditation is voluntary, and seeking deemed status through accreditation is an option, not a requirement. Accrediting bodies offer deemed status for various health care organizations across the continuum of care. Each accrediting body may accredit several types of health care organizations. While each accrediting body has to survey on the CMS CoPs, some accrediting bodies have chosen to create additional standards that organizations must adhere to.

Accreditation bodies include the following:

- The Joint Commission (TJC)

- National Integrated Accreditation of Healthcare Organizations (NIAHO) and ISO 9001 through Det Norske Veritas (DNV)

- Accreditation Association for Ambulatory Health Care Inc. (AAAHC)

- Community Health Accreditation Program (CHAP)

State Regulations and Regulating Agencies

Just as the federal government has a DHHS, each state has its own version as well. Some might be called HHS or just Department of Health. State health departments have different names and responsibilities: In some states, they are top-level administrative agencies, while in other states, they are a division or bureau of another office. Health departments are usually responsible for public health, including preventive medicine, epidemiology, vaccinations, environmental health (sometimes including health inspections), health statistics, developmental disabilities, mental health, occupational safety and health, receiving and recording reports of notifiable diseases, tobacco control, and the licensing of health care professionals. They are also responsible for collecting and archiving vital records such as birth and death certificates and sometimes marriage and divorce certificates.

In some states, state health departments may additionally be responsible for social services and welfare, environmental protection/pollution control, or the operation of the state psychiatric hospital (State Health Agencies, n.d.). At a more local level, in counties, parishes, boroughs, cities, and towns, there may be health care oversight for public health, community hospitals, and other organizations. Additionally, states manage health insurance through health care exchanges as part of the PPACA. There are so many differences in state oversight: It is important for you to visit your own state site and understand how they impact and drive health care in your state.

State Regulation of Professionals

Under the federal system of government in the US, each state regulates health care professionals' practice. Health professional practice acts are statutory laws that establish licensing or regulatory agencies or boards to generate rules that regulate practice. The major justification for regulating health professionals is to increase the quality of their services and thus to protect the public. Health professional regulations restrict entry into the profession by setting the minimum levels of education and experience required to practice. In addition, those regulations specify the legally permissible boundaries of practice for the nurse or provider.

Scope of practice, at minimum, is restricted to what the laws, rules, and regulations in your state permit based on what type of nurse or APRN you are. It is important that you read your scope of practice for the state in which you are licensed and practicing, as well as the scope of those you work with and those you staff and schedule. Effective and legal delegation cannot happen unless each licensed individual is aware of their own scope and what can or cannot be delegated to others. You can get to your state's and other states' nursing boards and nurse practice acts through an Internet search or via the National Council of State Boards of Nursing website (https://www.ncsbn.org/contactbon.htm).

More times than I prefer to hear, nurses confuse the role of their state board of nursing with a professional nursing association. The state board of nursing's main purpose is to regulate the profession of nursing to keep patients safe within the Nurse Practice Act. This includes setting the minimum standard for safe nursing care and determining the scope of practice for nurses within its jurisdiction while handling disciplinary actions for practice violations. The role of professional nursing associations such as the American Nurses Association is to advocate on behalf of nurses through establishing standards, scope of practice, and code of ethics. At the national and state levels, professional nursing organizations work to advance scope of practice and protect the practice of nursing.

Within our various health care systems, numerous organizations, accrediting bodies, and regulators influence our practice and care every day. We build policies and procedures to ensure our compliance; however, too few of us realize the full process, scope, and complexity of what drives patient care. As a nurse leading in the system, any system, it is vital you know the influences and, by all means, how you can be a part of the solution to influence and change them.

Key Points

- Outside the Medicare Part D expansion, the PPACA has been the largest piece of health care legislation since Medicare was originally created.

- As a nurse, you need to educate yourself about the PPACA so you can speak intelligently about it and educate others based on factual data.

- There are many ways to engage and make change happen at federal and national levels through various organizations.

- After congressional bills become laws, federal agencies are responsible for putting those laws into action through regulations or rules and need nurses' comments to drive best practices.

- The US health care system is very complex but manageable to navigate and change if you know the various organizations.

CHAPTER 3

What Is Systems Thinking?

When the number of factors coming into play
in a phenomenological complex is too large
scientific method in most cases fails.

One need only think of the weather,
in which case the prediction even for
a few days ahead is impossible.

—Albert Einstein

I love systems. I think in systems. To me everything is related somehow. Albert Einstein's quote reiterates our underdeveloped knowledge of organizations and systems and so much about the world we live in. This is also where chaos and complexity theory can help us come to a better understanding of the system.

This chapter is definitely more scientific and theoretical in nature. Do not worry; I do not want to lose anyone in this chapter. My goal is to discuss systems thinking, science, and theory in a manner you can understand and use in your own understanding of the world.

Systems Thinking

It has been said that everything is interconnected, but is that saying anything more substantial than a metaphor? Each similar industry is connected, but each different industry is also connected to other seemingly unrelated industries in ways that can be understood by micro- and macroeconomics. Health care is made up of many different industries and professions. Technology companies, banks, and academic institutions, as an example, are all interconnected and directly or indirectly impact the health care system. Therefore, they are part of the system like health insurance companies, hospitals, providers, and patients. And within each of these individual organizations, systems exist. It is helpful to think of industries and organizations as multilevel systems. Decades of research now exists to describe these multilevel systems at very high levels, as well as local levels. A basic understanding of systems and multilevel organizations is needed just to appreciate the complexity of the world you work and practice in, let alone create changes in it!

In chapters 1 and 2, system and health care system were defined. However, there is so much more detail to a system. There are many levels of systems: a cell, human body, animal packs, health care organizations, states, countries, and galaxies. All systems fall into one of two types: closed or open. Closed systems do not technically interact with and are considered isolated from the environment. Open systems do interact with the environment and have these components: output, feedback, input, and throughput (Haines, 1998).

Potentially the most important component in open systems, and therefore health care systems, is the ability to continuously import energy from the environment and export entropy (Wheatley, 2006). Often times, it is mistaken that open systems seek equilibrium, which is not true. Open systems that maintain a state of nonequilibrium keep themselves in a position to be able to change and grow (Wheatley, 2006). Structures that keep an open system growing include two different types of feedback loops, regulatory or negative and positive or amplifying feedback (Wheatley, 2006), which has led to the study of system dynamics. Disequilibrium is a necessary condition for a system to grow.

What happens when we fight change in the system? We ignore the negative feedback loop! Not changing and choosing stability over growth, will lead the organization and system to failure by ignoring the positive feedback loop. It is important to note that the positive feedback loop is not to be thought of as a pat on the back for a job well done. Quite the opposite! A positive or amplifying feedback loop uses information differently, not to regulate like a negative feedback loop but to notice something new in the environment that signals a need to change (Wheatley, 2006).

So what does a system have to do with nursing and health care? Everything! Health care systems have all the traits of an open system:

- The inputs are people needing care, the outputs are people cared for, and the feedback is the outcome measures, whether quality, financial, or patient satisfaction.

- There are numerous policies, procedures, and care guidelines in place to facilitate staff to be in a ready state to admit, discharge, transfer, and care for people despite the flu season or a catastrophic event.

- Each unit in a hospital has its own unique culture, different from the whole hospital, but contributing to the overall organization culture.

- Home health agencies or public health organizations have geographical boundaries for patients in which the organization may oversee in care.

- Regulations, accreditation standards, technology, and innovation provide inputs that we recognize as either negative or positive feedback.

A Little Organizational Theory

Starting in the late 1880s, along with the Industrial Revolution, the principles of scientific management, or Taylorism, appeared. This was the start in current thinking about managing organizations and employees, specifically to improve profits. Fredrick Taylor wanted to improve profits, so he did some of the first time and motion studies. This was the start of decades of organizational research. As people left farms and moved to the city for work, there was a growth in businesses and an apparent lack of understanding of human behavior within a system.

Business owners seeking to gain profits put little effort into the work environment and forced many workers to produce as much as they could without appropriate rewards. It is important to note that these were businesses prior to bureaucracy, which we will talk about later. These businesses were usually run by the owner and had no policies or procedures; thus, decisions such as hiring, work conditions, and firing were often made on the whim of the owner. There were no policies, procedures, or laws that protected employees, let alone standardized the equal treatment and pay of individuals. Many poor business practices led to the rise in unions and labor laws.

We also now have different schools of thought on management and human behavior in organizations, referred to as organizational theories.

As I discuss different theories and schools of thought, do not consider one better than another. As time has passed, we have learned things about organizations and have built on the prior knowledge to advance what we know now. What we learned in the early 1900s is still relevant today; however, it may be relevant in a different manner. One should never discount past knowledge and theories.

Taylorism, Time and Motion, and Nursing Care

Fredrick Taylor (1911) sought to improve worker efficiencies and commissioned many time and motion studies. These studies revolved around watching, timing, and improving on each step of a worker's process in order to improve efficiencies in manual labor. For instance, with a brick layer, how far did the brick layer have to reach to grab the next brick, and how long did it take to place the brick on the wall with mortar? To improve the efficiencies of a brick layer, the proximity of bricks would be improved so that the laborer did not have to spend more time than necessary reaching for one brick or retrieving supplies. By the mid-1900s, many other theories and schools of thought were generated from Taylor's work, mainly to address shortcomings. Criticism of Taylor's work included his lack of understanding of human behavior and its impact on work.

Today, while not called Taylorism, time and motion studies have been introduced in health care organizations in order to decrease waste and improve efficiencies. Nurses have demonstrated how time and motion studies are valuable even today. In a study performed across 36 hospitals, Chow et al. (2008) discovered that individual nurses traveled between 1 and 5 miles per 10-hour daytime shift and that nurses walked smaller distances during nighttime shifts when most activities and patient tasks decrease. The shape and layout of your unit do have an impact on how your staff functions, including their efficiency and effectiveness. If your organization is placing gel cleansing wall units up, with an expectation they are used, how much time and effort does it take for a nurse to walk to and use them? Time wasted in those activities takes away from directly caring for the patient.

Consider completing your own time and motion studies prior to engaging in a conversation for resources such as gel dispensers, computer work stations, and so on. It does not need to be a PhD-led research study. Engage your shared leadership or staff in completing this process improvement in data collection.

The Hawthorne Studies

Many people know the Hawthorne studies for the data from a 1924–1932 series of experiments at the Hawthorne Works, a General Electric factory near Chicago. The commissioned studies were devised to examine evidence that showed when workers think they are being watched, they produce better. The whole story is a little bit more than that. While we now know that Fredrick Taylor set the stage for many organizational studies, new researchers, wanting to expand on scientific management, decided to explore the effects of the organization's environment on the worker. Enter the Hawthorne studies, which initially looked at the effects of lighting on the worker, particularly which level of lighting improved productivity the most. The researchers also studied the effects of music, compensation, temperature, and hours worked.

What the researchers thought they discovered was the *experimenter effect*, sometimes called the observer effect. The experimenter effect is that the workers produced better outcomes regardless of the interventions. Why? The workers believed that because management was tinkering with the environment and making different changes, it was truly concerned with improving their work environment, worker satisfaction, and thereby productivity. It was not necessarily any one thing that improved individual productivity; it was the belief that management was concerned enough to continuously make improvements for them. (These studies have been extensively reexamined and debated ever since; Draper, 2013; Gale, 2004; Mostafazadeh-Bora, 2020.)

How many times have we implemented a change to improve staff satisfaction, only with the end result of no sustainable change? In the beginning, improvements are seen but taper off in the long run. Is it due to a lack of change management and embedding the change into the culture, or is it just the experimenter effect? It is important to base changes in your work environment on research, to actively use a change management process, and to measure your outcomes along the way! In some instances, scrapping a bad intervention early rather than continuing a change that is not valued might be the key to improving staff satisfaction.

Background on Bureaucracy

The word "bureaucracy" has become a bad word to many. When someone mentions the word "bureaucracy," it usually is in reference to a negative aspect of an organization and the inability to get things done. When Max Weber, a German sociologist, created his work on bureaucracies, he did not set out for this to be viewed negatively; rather, he believed that this was an ideal organizational structure. Essentially, a bureaucracy is a continuous system of authorized jobs maintained by regulations (Weber, 1968). The creation of bureaucracy was due in part to the business structures mentioned earlier, where there were no policies, procedures, or standards for business practices such as hiring, firing, and treating employees fairly. Think of bureaucracy as a stepping stone in the development of organizations. This structure, while maybe not the structure needed in today's environment, was a fundamental structural need when it was developed. This structure did help to advance the fundamental treatment of employees.

Two important features that add to the understanding of organizations were specialization and chain of command:

- *Specialization:* Encompasses a defined "sphere of competence" based on its divisions of labor

- *Chain of command:* In offices, a consistent organization of supervision based on distinctive levels of authority (Weber, 1968)

Bureaucracy is needed to create some form of organization; however, in an organization with professionals, this can lead to issues like negative perceptions of hierarchy. Cultures that are supportive of professional practice are built on the understanding that the essence of a professional model mandates that the privilege of autonomous practice be linked to the societal obligation to put the patient first. This obligation stems from an internal locus of control of the individual in the professional role that is supported by structure and process (Forsey & O'Rourke, 2013).

Instead of having high amounts of bureaucracy and hierarchy, professionals perform better when more control is within their professional ability to make their own decisions. Magnet hospitals build their structures on this premise and require a defined professional practice model (PPM) where professional role decision-making is clearly defined and supported (Forsey & O'Rourke, 2013).

Radical Management

Unfortunately, the intent of a bureaucracy has evolved to the point that it is perceived as negative and has come to stifle innovation and human spirit. We all feel like we are doing more with less and that if we just worked more and worked faster, things would be okay. That will never happen in a bureaucratic management structure. We cannot work harder and faster. Think about the 1960s, when Max Weber was outlining a bureaucratic structure. The world was quite a different place. Forward 30 years, with the Internet, equal access to knowledge, and globalization . . . as well as many industries shifting to an emphasis on customer satisfaction. If an organization or system wants to be or remain relevant, it will be hard to accomplish in a bureaucracy. So, how do we fix this? What is the next structure for today? How can we work smarter?

One consideration for today's structure is *radical management*. Denning (2010) notes that five shifts in today's structure need to take place. The five shifts must be undertaken simultaneously, and the result will be sustainable change that is radically more productive for the organization, more congenial to innovation, and more satisfying both for those doing the work and those for whom the work is done.

New Goal: From Inside-Out to Outside-In

Instead of telling the customer to take the services in the form that we provide, we need to listen to what the customer wants and provide them the service they want. And no, this does not make us a hotel and room service. If you have ever been a patient and received patient-centered care, you understand what this really means. And yes, there are patients that abuse this. But remember, the patient usually knows what they want from their health care experience.

New Role for Managers: From Controller to Enabler

It has been noted that there is a difference between managers and leaders. In a radical management system, managers MUST be leaders. Here, they must articulate goals, inspire change, and remove impediments. It is the workers—those doing the work—who get things done (Denning, 2010).

New Coordination: From Bureaucracy to Dynamic Linkage

Denning (2010) defines dynamic linking as a combination of four characteristics: (a) the work is done in short cycles; (b) the management sets the work goals for the cycle, based on what is known about patient experiences and outcomes;

(c) decisions about how the work should be carried out to achieve those goals are largely the responsibility of those doing the work; and (d) progress is measured by direct client feedback through surveys and patients and families on hospital committees. This sounds a lot like shared leadership. When I hear that shared governance does not work in an organization, often its due to the managers holding on to traditional bureaucratic management where they default to controlling individuals. In radical management, the management must move from controller to enabler. Dynamic linking can not occur within radical management by skipping steps. Those who are closest to the work need to be the ones who decide how it gets done.

From Value to Values

In traditional organizations, the focus is on value and profit, even at the expense of the customer or patient (Denning, 2010). In a values-based organization, the focus is shifted toward positive customer experience. With the increase in transparency from public reporting of quality and satisfaction measures, the public can see the results of the management of a health care organization. Are they value or values based? This does not mean a company cannot make a profit. In fact, research shows a radical management structure is two to four times more productive than traditional teams.

Radical management is way of managing an organization that generates at the same time high productivity, continuous innovation, high job satisfaction, and high customer satisfaction (Denning, 2011).

Communications: From Command to Conversation

A lot of literature speaks about how to deal with the younger generations. Most of this focuses on communication, decreased hierarchy, and a human-to-human

A CONSIDERATION FOR SYSTEMS THINKING	
In 2009, Hartmann et al. found that higher levels of safety climate were significantly associated with higher amounts of group and entrepreneurial culture, while lower amounts of safety climate were associated with higher	levels of hierarchical cultures. This is an important finding in that professional practice models by their nature require less hierarchy and more autonomy to clinical decision-making, collaboration, and transparency (Loos & O'Rourke, 2012).

approach. This is interesting as it is called for in the fifth change for a radical management approach. In order to make this successful shift, there needs to be a shift in the mode of communication from command to conversation, with adult-to-adult interactions, using stories, metaphors, and open-ended questions (Denning, 2010). Regardless of what generation one is working with (which is probably all four), successful communication is carried out predominantly through the language of social norms. Pushback will occur in organizations where relationships are dominated by hierarchy (Denning, 2010).

As you continue to read about other theories and the macro and micro levels of organizations and systems, it should become clearer why organizations and systems choose to remain bureaucracies, which is an attempt to control the complexity. However, it should also be clear why that is not the right answer for leading in the system.

There are many organizational theories and behavioral theories. Each theory describes different phenomena that are used to study and explain organizations and systems. Organizational theories are useful in explaining and helping to resolve issues. I encourage all individuals to continue to read more about various organizational and management theories. I have also included other theories in other chapters based on the topics. Theories will not always give you answers but will help guide you to think broadly about leading!

Modern Theories

General Systems Theory

General systems theory (GST) has evolved over several decades, but the main point of this theory is that the whole is greater than the sum of its parts. Many nurses may have heard that point made, and often it is assumed to be metaphorical in nature. GST at the micro and macro levels should be considered much more than a metaphor in organizational science. Further discussion about macro and micro will occur a little later in this chapter.

Systems theorists had a goal to create a general systems theory that explained everything about systems in all fields of science. Ludwig von Bertalanffy was just one of the early systems theorists but is most often credited with the creation of GST. In GST, it has been theorized that general system laws exist that apply to any system of a certain type, irrespective of the particular properties of the system and the elements involved. It is not a theory of management but a theory to assist with conceptualizing an organization in a new and different way and understanding emergence (discussion on emergence will come later in this chapter). GST seeks to expand the ability in which individuals examine and understand organizational behavior. There are two types of systems referred to by GST: open systems and closed systems (see below). An open system is an organization that interacts with other organizations outside of itself, and a closed system is an organization that has little interaction with others outside of itself. The principles of open systems are as follows:

- Parts that make up the system are interrelated

- Health of overall system is contingent on subsystem functioning

- Open systems import and export material from and to the environment

- Permeable boundaries

- Relative openness

- Second principle of thermodynamics

  - Entropy must increase to a maximum

  - Negentropy increases growth and a state of survival

- Synergy (whole is greater than sum of parts)

- Equifinality versus "one best way"

The principles of closed systems are the following:

- Do not recognize they are embedded in a relevant environment

- Overly focused on internal functions and behaviors

- Do not recognize or implement equifinality

- Inability to use feedback appropriately

- Codependent versus interdependent

Nursing leaders need to understand their organization's position in reference to the open–closed system continuum. While no organization is truly a closed unit, department, or system in our current culture, it may not be as open to the environment as it needs to be to maximize functioning. As a nursing leader, what can you do to help maximize functioning and partner with the environment to enhance patient care?

Chaos Theory

Many individuals have not heard of chaos theory but have heard of the butterfly effect. There is even a movie named after this phenomenon. This theory describes how the smallest change can have a large impact; for example, the flapping of a butterfly's wings in one part of the world could cause a hurricane half a world away. Here, something very simple (such as the flapping of the butterfly's wings) leads to a much more complex outcome that cannot be predicted solely by looking at the parts of the whole. Just like in complexity theory, we see that patient care consists of numerous processes in which multiple factors or agents exert influence on availability, application, and sequence in highly variable ways, which results in outcomes that are less than fully predictable. Due to the multiple factors we know and do not know, the decisions we make can impact things that we never intended to change.

Complexity Theory

Complexity theory is based on physics and has been applied in the field of organizational science. Complexity theory is a loose set of concepts, heuristics (educated guess, intuition, common sense, etc.), and analytic tools. The most important understanding to take away from complexity theory is that relationships are the key to everything (Wheatley, 2006). Key concepts of complexity theory are dissipative systems, patterns, and attractor.

Quite often, individuals confuse complexity theory and chaos theory or even consider them one and the same. While they are both considered nonlinear systems, they are different. Complexity theory refers to systems that are made up of a large number of parts and their interactions. Chaos theory can have a small number of interacting parts. Chaos theory is based on the geometrical mathematical principle of fractals.

Weather is a complex pattern. It seems random and unpredictable, but while we cannot always predict with 100 percent accuracy the exact temperature for a certain day, we can know for certain if it will be warm or cold. This is like health care, where there are many seemingly random patterns and components. Patient care consists of numerous processes with multiple factors that influence availability, application, and sequence in highly variable ways, which results in outcomes that are less than fully predictable. As we talk later about data and applying certain practices to patients, recognize that even with the best data, it is impossible to be 100 percent accurate in predicting patient outcomes as we do not have all the components influencing the outcomes. As a nurse leader, be aware of the complexity of everything in your unit, department, or system. Seek to learn about the things you do not know, such as the micro and macro perspectives that we will discuss later in this chapter.

Complex Adaptive and Emergent Systems

A complex adaptive system in healthcare can be defined as "when the parts (in the case of the U.S. health care system, this includes human beings) have the freedom and ability to respond to stimuli in many different and fundamentally unpredictable ways. For this reason, emergent, surprising, creative behavior is a real possibility" (IOM, 2001 p. 310). Within a complex adaptive emergent (CAS), a system is part of a larger system that is organized in a fractal manner. A fractal is a geometric shape that can be separated into parts, each of which is a reduced-scale version of the whole (Mandelbrot, 2008). There are many examples in nature of a fractal, including seashells, snowflakes, lightning, trees, the human circulatory system, health care systems, and even that head of Romanesco broccoli. In these examples, fractals have similar patterns that recur at progressively smaller scales. Fractal categories include nature, computers, math, time, physical structures, time, sound, and art, for example.

A world patterned in fractals does not explain itself through traditional measures (Wheatley, 2006). Here, we must focus on qualitative measures as opposed to only a very quantitative, objective, measurable world. As noted in chapter 2, we have many organizations that collect, measure, and report the data of our health system in order to improve it. "Instead of gaining clarity, our search for quantification leads us into infinite fogginess. The information never ends, and it is never complete, we accumulate more and more but understand less and less. Deep inside the details, we cannot see the whole. Yet, to understand and work with the system, we need to be able to observe it as a system, in its wholeness. Wholeness is revealed only as shapes, not facts. Systems reveal themselves as patterns, not as isolated incidents or data points" (Wheatley, 2006, p. 125).

In understanding the context of an organization, look for patterns, which are anything that happens more than once. Do not try to reduce the pattern, looking for isolated factors or individuals that may be involved. Ask yourself questions like the following:

- Have we seen this before?

- What feels familiar here?

In order to understand the patterns, we must step back as shapes are not discerned from close range (i.e., looking for a reductionist answer) (Wheatley, 2006). Patterns in organizations are often explained as the culture of an organization.

Fractal systems have many proprieties. One important property is emergence. Emergence is the phenomenon of agents interacting within the system in what looks like random ways as opposed to planned or controlled. From all these interactions, patterns emerge, informing the behavior of both individuals and the system. By observing the behavior of a nurse or senior executive, you can see what the organization values and how it chooses to express what it appreciates (Wheatley, 2006), and the culture, good or bad, emerges.

Multilevel Thinking

Macro and Micro Perspectives

When thinking about systems, I want you to think about both the macro and the micro perspectives of organizations. Organizations are too complex to only think about one perspective and make a sustainable change. So, what type of thinking brings both together? Multilevel thinking. *Multilevel thinking* brings together the macro and micro perspectives. Often, one might see a focus around one or the other, but to understand, appreciate, and make meaningful changes in an organization, both perspectives need to be at the table!

Multilevel thinking is complex. I hear you saying, "I can barely keep track of what is going on in my own department already!" But it is usually unnecessarily complex because one does not fully appreciate or know both the perspectives that are occurring in an organization. Decisions, many wrong, are made based on only one perspective of an organization or the system.

In order to change health care at our local and national levels, each of us needs to become an expert in our systems thinking so we can lead in our system! Keep in mind: "The primary goal of the multilevel perspective in organizational science is to identify principles that enable a more integrated understanding of phenomena that unfold across all levels in organizations" (Klein & Kozlowski, 2000, p. 7). As a nurse, you need to understand enough about both perspectives to ask meaningful questions and make sustainable changes.

The Macro Perspective

The macro perspective on organizations is rooted in sociology and holds that there are enough similarities among individuals that aggregated data or averages about groups can be used and individual variations can be ignored. This plays out in several ways in a health care organization and for nurses.

There is a danger inherent in the macro perspective, which is thinking that organizations "behave." They do not; people do. Macro-level data typically ignore the ways in which individual behavior, perceptions, and interactions develop and impact higher-level phenomena (Klein & Kozlowski, 2000).

There are reasons why a nurse may want or not want to aggregate data (table 3.1). This is not by any means saying that you should use the data that make your department look best. I am saying that you should know not only your data but also the source. Know when they should be aggregated and when they should not be. Understand that aggregated data are made up of micro-level occurrences. Many times, organizations take aggregated data and attempt to apply them to a lower level. What detail is lost when you look at the averages, and can you really arrive at a full understanding of an issue when using aggregated data?

In research class, everyone learns about the "generalizability" of a study. When performing research, the goal is to be able to generalize quantitative research results

---

A CONSIDERATION FOR SYSTEMS THINKING

Using Macro-level Data

A particular department's patient satisfaction data are typically aggregated to a "macro" level, meaning there is an average number given for a satisfaction ranking. Remember that one patient for whom no nurse or staff member could do any good? They are in that aggregated data, and what is bad is that their low scoring survey pulls the department's overall score down. Is this an accurate reflection of the overall care provided by staff? Furthermore, can you imagine getting 50 individual surveys with no data aggregation? How would you know if your department was improving overall? If there was an issue, how would you be able to trend issue data? Aggregated data are useful in certain situations within the appropriate context.

Do not fall into the trap of blindly accept aggregated data without knowing the details in the aggregation.

Table 3.1. Considerations for Using Macro-Level Data

BENEFITS	POTENTIAL ISSUES
Less data to look at	Individual variations are ignored
Data are in an average format	Data can be inappropriately interpreted
Benchmarking is easier	Action plans may not address genuine issues
Data can be compared across departments	Real issue with an individual may be masked
Standardized action plans can be created	May be a misspecification of error

upward and outward. The results obtained are considered applicable to others for use and incorporation into practice. But in qualitative research, we learn that you really cannot generalize results to other groups. The main thought on why qualitative research cannot be generalized is that an individual's response is based on their worldview and context, and each person has a unique context that would get lost in a quantitative attempt to generalize.

There is a similar issue to consider with macro-level data, called misspecification. This occurs when an organization takes aggregated data and attempts to generalize the data downward to lower levels in an organization, assuming they apply. They do not. Why not? Each lower level has its unique culture that may not be reflected by the aggregated data from the higher macro level.

How does this apply to your department? How many times did the organizations or the corporate office take aggregated data, create an action plan, and give it to individual departments to carry out, assuming this was going to make some positive change? Too many times for any of us to count. Quite often, this method failed and the blame was placed on an individual instead of a failed process and belief system.

Lesson? Do not create an action plan based on high-level aggregated data with the hope of rolling out the action plan to local departments with an expectation for successful change without some understanding. You and your organization might be committing an act of misspecification!

The Micro Perspective

On the flip side is the micro perspective on organizations, which concerns itself with the individual or lower levels of an organization. It is important to remember that despite the micro perspective being about individuals or lower levels, it is not immune to the context of the higher levels of an organization. In the macro

Table 3.2. Considerations for Using Micro-Level Data

BENEFIT	POTENTIAL ISSUES
Individual variations understood	Too much data to make an interpretation
Unique specific action plans created	Unable to determine benchmark
Individuals treated as individuals	Loss of ability to compare across units or departments
Specific concerns addressed	Atomistic fallacy

perspective, I discussed the issues with assuming the higher levels of the organization always reflect the lower levels; however, that is not to say that higher levels of the organization have no effect on lower levels or vice versa.

Just as potential issues with misspecification occur in macro-level thinking, there are also errors in thinking at the micro level. Improvements within an individual do not necessarily translate into improvements at a higher macro level. An assumption of this type can cause an error called an atomistic fallacy. An atomistic fallacy occurs when erroneous inferences are made about causal relationships in aggregate units based on data measured at individual levels (Diez Roux, 2002).

It is important to note that just because an organizational intervention was based on individual data does not always mean it ends in failure. This means that leaders need to understand that failure can occur when making decisions that involve individual-level data. Table 3.2 notes considerations for using micro-level data.

Top-Down and Bottom-Up in Systems Thinking

Organizations are too complex to think that a process or event in one unit has no effect on the whole organization. Similarly, the larger organization can also influence lower levels of the organization. Which way do we go? We go the meso way. *Meso* is the term used by organizational scientists to describe an integrated approach in considering both the micro and macro perspectives. This is a multilevel approach to systems thinking.

Top-Down Processes

Top-down processes refer to contextual influences; that is, each level of an organization and each organization, for that matter, are embedded within larger organizations or systems. A unit or department is part of an organization. An organization such as a clinic or hospital is a part of a chain or group of clinics or hospitals. A group of hospitals and clinics is a part of an accountable care organization (ACO). An ACO is part of the US health care system.

A top-down process refers to the influence of higher-level contextual factors on lower levels of the system (Klein & Kozlowski, 2000). Contextual factors are characteristics of the environment. For instance, an organization determines rules (such as when employees come to work or the chain of command) for employees related to human resource processes. These types of rules that have a direct impact on the employee can help determine the culture of the organization. If there is a highly bureaucratic process for making changes, individual employees could see this as a negative culture, and it would have a negative impact on employees trying to effect change.

Similarly, the US health care system has processes and rules in place for provider and organizational reimbursement. Individual organizations create departments and processes in response to higher-level rules to get paid. The perception of the organization could be that the US health care system is full of regulations. These factors all create processes that move from the top down into each level below.

Bottom-Up Processes

Bottom-up processes are also considered emergent. This describes how lower-level properties emerge to form collective phenomena (Klein & Kozolowski, 2000). This is where individual- or lower-level phenomena impact the culture of higher levels. For instance, a leader in a department can have a negative effect on the morale of employees. In turn, employees leave the organization, other departments hear of poor morale, and their fear for their own department creates a culture of poor morale and decreased staff satisfaction across the organization.

Emergence

As we learned earlier, emergence has its foundation in GST, chaos, and complexity theories, as well as a core property of fractal systems. There is even a term (*emergent complexity*) that refers to the belief that the organization develops from the bottom up and can be explained by very complex patterns. Emergence attempts to understand how dynamics and interactions of lower-level phenomena occur over time to create structure or process phenomena at a higher level (Klein & Kozlowski, 2000). There are two types of emergence: compilation and composition. These two types of emergence are important in your use of data every day! Make sure you understand these two types. As I discuss these two types, think about the data you use, how you make decisions based on the data, and how you might use the data differently based on whether they are a compilation or a composition in nature.

Compilation

Compilation is based on the "assumption of discontinuity and describes phenomena that comprise a common domain but are distinctively different as they emerge across levels" (Klein & Kozlowski, 2000, p. 16). An example might be the concept of professionalism. This concept is functionally equivalent at both the unit and organizational levels; however, it is not an identical concept at each of those levels. This can occur because lower-level characteristics, behaviors, and perceptions may vary within each group and influence the antecedents and processes at every level (Klein & Kozlowski, 2000). The antecedents (which are defined as things that come before something else) of professionalism for an individual RN are not all the same as the antecedents of professionalism for the organization.

Composition

Composition is based "on the assumptions of isomorphism, which describes phenomena that are essentially the same as they emerge upwards across levels" (Klein & Kozlowski, 2000, p. 16). Composition is different from compilation in that here, the concept of service at the individual level could be the same concept with the same antecedents at a higher level.

To add to any confusion you may have, sometimes a phenomenon could be a composition and the same phenomenon could be a compilation depending on the circumstances. Let us look at professionalism as the concept. The professionalism of an individual RN can influence or change the concept of professionalism at the unit or department level. However, professionalism at the unit or department level may have an impact on individual RN professionalism as well. When you are creating an action plan to resolve an issue, here are some examples of questions you should consider (picking professionalism as the phenomenon here, but any concept will work):

- What does this concept mean to your department as a whole?

- What does this mean to each nurse?

- Are there nurses who may have more influence in creating a different perception (which is a different definition) of professionalism for the department as a whole?

- What type of action plan is really most appropriate? An individual specific action plan or an action plan for the whole department?

- Is the creation of a department-wide action plan really more about you as a leader not wanting to address the behavior of a few individuals that is creating havoc at the department level?

When working with your unit, department, or organization, it is important to understand that the phenomena with which you work daily are either from a top-down or bottom-up process. Furthermore, those processes can affect how you make changes and lead your unit.

Ecological Fallacy

An ecological fallacy is to "conclude that a positive cross-sectional correlation between a specific operational practice and performance implies that implementing the practice will improve performance" (Ketokivi et al., 2021, p. 2070). For example, you receive your employee engagement scores. Overall, you did better than average, but on recognition, you were slightly below average, and you will need to complete an action plan on this one item. You schedule a forum to talk to staff about how you can improve recognition. However, having a group forum may be due to a logical fallacy in your data interpretation. You realize that the individuals who probably scored you the lowest might not come to discuss their reasons one on one, but having a group forum assumes that each individual who attends scored you the same as your average, when in fact you probably had a mix: some may have scored you average, you might have had some higher scores, and then you must have had some individuals score you low.

This does not mean you do not get to complete an action plan, but you do need to think about what the data are really saying and how you can create a meaningful action plan to improve your scores. Instead of a group forum to understand why the group scored you below average (as we know now, the entire group may not have), as you meet with each individual staff member (hopefully, something you do on a routine basis), ask them how they like to be recognized. This takes the

Working with the Culture at All Levels

While traversing countries, universities, and health care systems during my career, I have garnered some firsthand perspectives about optimizing opportunities and overcoming obstacles within organizations. An overarching insight stems from understanding the culture of the organization by observing the institutional commitment demonstrated by those working in the system, whatever their role or position.

Within a week of arriving in the US from England, I found myself in charge of a busy transitional care unit in a county hospital. I called for a "porter to get a trolley to take the patient in the lift to the theater." As soon as I heard "A who for what on the what to where?" I realized I needed help. A "translator" told me I needed to ask for an orderly to get a gurney to take the patient in the elevator to the operating room. I learned fast that it is important to use the right language in the context of the environment. What took longer to understand, however, was the gap I heard identified between "us and them" (them being the richer hospitals). Our culture was to belittle ourselves, to save pushing for excellence for other hospitals, to be satisfied just getting through on a day-to-day basis.

This troubled me and became a catalyst for powerful, unbiased, multilevel conversations, which concentrated on what we did well and why we had so much to be proud of—namely, our outstanding patient care. We did not need the frills of wallpaper and single rooms; we needed each other and pride in what we knew we did well. Many years later, I discovered this process was coined appreciative inquiry—discovering what works well in any situation, capitalizing on existing strengths, and adjusting the sails as needed. Being involved in shaping a system's culture is an opportunity for employees at all levels of the organization to measure personal success in terms of impact rather than status. One example where I witnessed unparalleled commitment is shared governance. I chaired a system research council involving three distant hospitals. Despite environmental and staffing differences, we set a dedicated focus to reporting and sharing best practices. From this came published research, which reached institutional attention from the bedside to the boardroom—calming practices in preoperative care that greatly improved patient satisfaction. This cascaded to nurses empowering each other to ensure evidence-based practice became a part of the institutional culture.

Miki Goodwin, PhD, RN, PH

pressure off of them for a perceived shortcoming in your leadership skills while allowing them to express how they prefer to be recognized. Then you will have a meaningful action plan based on individuals giving you their individual perception. Remember, for some staff, you were probably doing the right things already in recognizing them! What you do not want to do is to shift away from doing the right things with those staff members and layer on one or several recognition initiatives that a few people suggest or are only meaningful to some.

Organizational theories and other theories are useful in broadening our perspective about the systems and organizations in which we work and live. Often these theories do not provide answers but guide us to seek answers that are right for our departments and organizations.

Key Points

- Health care systems are open systems.

- Bureaucracy is needed to create some form of organization.

- Radical management is a structure that truly supports shared leadership.

- Think about both the macro and the micro perspective of organizations.

- Build an action plan that is meaningful to individuals and does not layer additional work on top of everything people are doing.

CHAPTER 4
Innovation and Standardization

Never doubt that a small group of thoughtful,
committed citizens can change the world.
Indeed, it's the only thing that ever has.

—Margaret Mead

The US is known for some amazing innovations, forward-thinking technology, and great scientists. If you need great medical equipment and the best of the new surgical methods to save your life, you are in the right country. But the problem is that we will save you only to possibly harm or kill you through system errors during your hospitalization, through an error or lack of communication in the care transition to the home care agency, or by not talking with your primary care provider. Medical errors are the third leading cause of death in the US, with new estimates as high as 400,000 per year (Makary & Daniel, 2016), significantly higher than that of the 1999 Institute of Medicine (IOM) *To Err Is Human* report. None of this is intentional, but it is a result of watching and not managing feedback closer in our care delivery models.

One way we can change the system is to lead innovation and standardization at the same time! This may seem like an oxymoron. How can you have innovation and be standardized? For many, standardization is a concept far from innovation. Once we standardize something, we can leave it alone for years and not have to worry about it. We all strive to get take things off our to do lists, celebrate finishing something, and move on to the next issue. But that is the problem. We cannot completely move on from anything.

Standardization does not stifle innovation if we build in feedback loops and continue to monitor for when it does need to be changed. We need both standardization and innovation at the same time. The key is to have a process for innovation, a process for when and how to standardize, and a process that always allows that standardization to be updated, tested, and innovated upon quickly.

Quite often the issue of innovation and standardization is change. We will talk more about change and the problems with change in the next chapter. In this chapter, I am going to discuss innovation and standardization: what they are and how and why you need to bring the two together!

Innovation in Health Care Organizations

Over the past several years, health care organizations have been navigating through unprecedented times: months and years of budget shortfalls, staffing shortages, and personal protective equipment and equipment shortages due to the COVID-19 pandemic. The pandemic has increased many organizations' bad debt, decreased revenue, and increased expenses. In many organizations, important initiatives and innovations were placed on hold due to the uncertainty, and in others, programs and staff were cut as one answer to weathering these changes.

It is well known and accepted that innovation is a major driver of increases in medical spending due to higher utilization (Baker et al., 2003; Newhouse, 1992). One reason is that the innovation tends to have low as opposed to high productivity (Cahan et al., 2020). The following are examples of low and high productivity (Cahan et al., 2020).

LOW PRODUCTIVITY	HIGH PRODUCTIVITY
Additive to Patient Care	Substitutive to Patient Care
Business Model Sustaining	Business Model Disrupting
Content Based	Process Based

Nursing innovation has been in both low- and high-productivity buckets but remains mostly additive and content based. The health care system has tried a few times to move into high-productivity innovation due to changes in federal legislation. Through the 1990s, after the 1983 change from fee for service to the prospective payment system (PPS), organizations cut costs where they could, often through staff layoffs, without changing the model of care and with insufficient focus on process. And now, since 2010 and the Affordable Care Act (ACA), the Center for Medicare & Medicaid Innovation (CMMI) has launched over 40 new payment models looking toward process-based innovations that drive cost savings and improve care. So far, only two programs, the Diabetes Prevention Program (DPP) model and the Pioneer ACO model, have met the requirements to be cost savings but have yet to be made part of the full Medicare program.

Innovation is often thought of as some radical or brand-new idea or concept, like something futuristic from a *Star Trek* movie or rerun. Innovation can be that, but it can also be a recombining of current and seemingly disparate ideas that result in something new. Even a different use for something that has been around 50 years can be innovation! Innovation can be anywhere on the continuum of incremental to radical (Scott & Mensik, 2010). When you think innovation, think science and technology. To have innovation, you must have both. A great piece of knowledge does not mean much unless we can translate it into use.

A good idea before its time is a bad idea, even with innovation. I liken this to the use of telehealth in home health patients. In a program I oversaw in the mid-2000s, we decreased the readmission rates for over 500 New York Heart Association (NYHA) stage 2 and 3 patients to only 3 percent in a 12-month period. Only 3 percent of patients were readmitted for heart failure in a year. Great for the patient, but bad for the bottom line. Hospitals and nurses depended on people being sick. We wanted patients to stay out of the hospital but not stay out too long. Now that we have the Patient Protection and Accountable Care Act and account-able care with a focus on prevention, we may start to see changes that shift that thinking. The point is not to stop innovating if there are barriers but continue to lead in the system to make the changes that are best for our patients!

The conventional delivery of health care services, such as stand-alone organiza-tions, can no longer stand up to the combined forces of market fluctuations, health care financing, new technologies, and the aging population. The typical response from many hospital and health care organization administrators is that they cannot afford to innovate and change during such an uncertain time, even more so on the heels of the pandemic. But we need nurses, health care organizations, and systems to drive process-based, high-productivity solutions. Even with all the uncertainty that will always exist, there is never a "good" or "best" time to change. It is important to note that research and history show that companies that invest in their innovative capabilities during tough economic times are those that fare best when growth returns (Chesbrough & Garman, 2009). To invest in innovation and change, many organizations have or will merge or be acquired by larger health care systems to survive in the long term.

The Difference between Knowledge Generation and Translation

To lead change, we all need to know the differences and definitions. Science is a "knowledge or a system of knowledge covering general truths, or the operation of general laws especially as obtained and tested through scientific method" (Merriam-Webster, n.d.). Science generates, synthesizes, and accumulates knowledge in one narrow area; its models hold much else "fixed." On the other hand, technology is the search for and production of theories about new processes. Technology is the application of existing knowledge; its models allow most everything to vary. Simply put, science is the "why" while technology is the "how" of improvement (Szczerba & Huesch, 2012, p. 103). This is why we can be innovative, as technology allows us to use and apply what we learned in science in different ways.

The translation or application of knowledge (i.e., technology) remains far less funded and less visible than the generation, synthesis, and accumulation of knowledge (i.e., science), and the two are only weakly integrated. Worse, technology is often seen merely as an adjunct to practice (e.g., electronic health records). For example, the electronic health records and process control do not capture the full potential of what technology can offer. By integrating existing knowledge from behavioral science, organization science, engineering, and clinical research and applying this in simulated environments, technology can improve and redesign existing care processes as well as engineer new ones (Szczerba & Huesch, 2012, p. 103).

In nursing, we have acknowledged the need for both research and translation. Thus, our profession has both the PhD in Nursing and a Doctorate of Nursing Practice (DNP) degree. The DNP degree is considered the knowledge translation degree, whereas the PhD is considered the knowledge generator or researcher degree. For decades, we have graduated PhD-prepared nurses who have generated great knowledge but did not have doctorally prepared RNs to assist in the translation into practice. Thus, much of that knowledge has stayed in textbooks and peer-reviewed journals.

Various studies have shown that it takes 17 to 20 years to get clinical innovations into practice and, worse, that fewer than 50 percent of clinical innovations ever make it into general usage (Bauer & Kirchner, 2020). It is also estimated that 80 percent of medical research dollars do not make an impact on public health (Chalmers & Glasziou, 2009) for various reasons. More than half a million new items of biomedical research are generated every year and added to Medline (a database of medical publications). We are not very good at applying this steady accumulation of scientific knowledge and thereby improving health care in the United States (Szczerba & Huesch, 2012, p. 103).

Often, we have a system that overvalues local autonomy and undervalues disciplined science (recall my quote about autonomy nuts by Dr. Lucian Leape). Our inability to incorporate new knowledge in practice is not because of inattention or incompetence among doctors and nurses but because it is difficult for the human mind to keep up with the explosion of knowledge (Swenson et al., 2010).

Setting the Stage for Innovation

As with other sections of this book, this chapter is not immune to theory and theory application. There are many theories one can use for innovation; however, I will not bore you with them all, indulging you in only one: the diffusion of innovation.

Diffusion of Innovation

The process in which an innovation moves is referred to as innovation diffusion. Many researchers have noted that this process of diffusion is predictable regardless of the innovation. Diffusion of innovation is a theory that seeks to explain

---

A CONSIDERATION FOR SYSTEMS THINKING

An Innovative Insight

As you are reading about innovation, knowledge generation, and translation, think about the following quote from Dr. Farzad Mostashari: "Data is the oxygen of innovation" (Mostashari, 2014). We will discuss the importance of data in chapter 8.

how, why, and at what rate new ideas and technology spread (Rogers, 2003). The theory was first discussed in the book *Diffusion of Innovations*, written by Everett Rogers and first published in 1962. It has been well received and is now in its fifth edition. Rogers states that diffusion is the process by which an innovation is communicated through certain channels over time among the members of a social system. The theory states that four main elements influence the spread of a new idea:

- The innovation

- Communication channels

- Time

- A social system (Rogers, 2003)

This influence relies heavily on human capital. The innovation must be widely adopted to self-sustain. Within the rate of adoption, there is a point at which an innovation reaches critical mass. The categories of adopters (table 4.1) are innovators, early adopters, early majority, late majority, and laggards (Rogers, 2003). Which adopter category do you fit in related to your personal or professional life?

Table 4.1. Diffusion of Innovation as Applied to the Smartphone

ADOPTER CATEGORY	RATE OF ADOPTION (PERCENT)	DEFINITION
Innovators	2.5	The first individuals to adopt an innovation: These individuals have latest version of technology and will be the first people walking around with Google Glass (wearable computer that displays information like a smartphone but hands-free).
Early adopters	13.5	Get the latest version of technology once they determine it is "safe"; they try out new things and they are opinion leaders.
Early majority	34	Will purchase the technology but are thoughtful and careful; they adopt change before the majority.
Late majority	34	Finally get some version of the technology once the majority is using it; they are skeptical.
Laggards	16	Still own the old technology (or maybe none at all) and do not see need for new technology. May only adopt once it is a tradition or they are forced into it, whichever comes first.

The theory also states that innovations are adopted by organizations through two types of innovation decisions: collective innovation decisions and authority innovation decisions. The collective innovation decision occurs when the adoption of an innovation has been made by a consensus among the members of an organization. "The authority innovation-decision occurs when the adoption of an innovation has been made by very few individuals with high positions of power within an organization" (Rogers, 2003, p. 403). Within the innovation decision process in an organization, there are certain individuals, called "champions," who stand behind an innovation and break through any opposition that the innovation may have caused.

The champion or change agent becomes important not just to manage the change but to create that shared vision and provide the leadership that will sustain the innovation until it is self-sustaining. It is believed that once it has been adopted by approximately 15 percent of individuals, the diffusion process is irreversible. The structures and processes by which innovations may become self-sustaining could be policies, procedures, standards of care, education, and job descriptions in an organization. The champion ensures that the vision and the intent of the innovation are not lost in translation or, more important, not lost because "our patients are different here."

Design Thinking and Hackathons

Nurses have always been innovators. How many times have you needed to problem solve an issue, jerry-rigging the solution with tubing, tape, or equipment so that care could be given? Despite this, nurses usually do not think of themselves as innovators (Kagan et al., 2021). Yet, nurses are perfect for being innovators. The nursing process has given us all a head start in how to think and solve unique issues.

Design thinking and hackathons go hand in hand. First, what is design thinking? Design thinking is a methodology to generate innovative solutions through creative problem solving. It is nonlinear and iterative. There are a few schools of thought on the components of design thinking. One of the most popular views includes the five components based on the Interaction Design Foundation:

- Empathy—gain insight into the user and their needs

- Define—state the problem in a human-centered manner

- Ideate—identify innovative solutions to the problem defined

- Prototype—decide on the best possible solution

- Test—test solutions to understand product and users (Interaction Design Foundation, 2020)

Hackathons

So, what is a hackathon? "Hackathons are organized to bring together both experienced and novice individuals from a variety of backgrounds to brainstorm creative solutions to complex issues" (Mevawala et al., 2021, p. E154).

In the past decade, nurse-led hackathons, incubators, and accelerators have emerged to meet for a formalized process for nurses to gather to solve issues facing them every day (Kagan et al., 2021). Numerous organizations have held events for hackathons as well as podcasts telling the stories of nurse innovators:

- Johnson & Johnson Nurse Innovation Hackathons https://nursing.jnj.com /nurse-innovation-hackathons

- See You Now ANA and Johnson & Johnson podcasts

- Amplify Nursing Penn Nursing podcasts

Standardization in Health Care Organizations

The connection between quality in health care and standardization is similar to an observation by psychologist Erich Fromm (1956): "Just as modern mass production requires the standardization of commodities, so the social process requires standardization of man, and this standardization is called equality" (p. 78). Standardization allows health care providers to provide equality in care, one of the components in the IOM's definition of quality. According to the online Merriam-Webster dictionary, standardization means "to change (things) so that they are similar and consistent and agree with rules about what is proper and acceptable," and as evidence based practice (EBP) is the process that determines what to standardize, we need to put this knowledge into a form we can use. These forms may include policies, procedures, standards of care, and clinical decision support systems.

With the explosion of knowledge as allowed through the creation and use of the Internet and World Wide Web, we have chaos, which leads some to constructive action. This is where wise standardization is a foundation for effective variation, efficiency, reliability, and rapid innovation (Swensen et al., 2010). After a process is stable, we can more effectively eliminate waste that does not add value. Humans working in a standardized environment are supported in achieving higher reliability. Standardization facilitates the assessment of the comparative effectiveness of interventions by providing a baseline against which potential improvements can be measured (Swensen et al., 2010).

Standardizing policies, procedures, and other such documents is no easy task in one department, and it is tougher across units or organizations, especially if you are not used to doing things this way. But it is very possible! This is how you will ensure the evidence is placed into practice and used. When we look at the inefficiencies in health care, how many times as nurses did we feel the need to create our own policies for something on our unit when they already existed on another unit or at another facility? What could we have been doing with that time that would have served the patients better?

Standardization should occur in policies, procedures, standards of care, and processes across organizations. And it can. The usual pushback excuse is "but our patients are different," which is usually not the case. There may be many factors that are different, but this is where wise standardization occurs. Policies and procedures should not get into the details of every step of the process but outline the expected steps and actions that are evidence based.

A CONSIDERATION FOR SYSTEMS THINKING

Adopting Innovation

Many times I have heard people say, get one of the naysayers on your side and you will have no problem making a change! This method does work. But think about the innovation curve. The naysayers, by definition, are not the innovators or early adopters. And it is important to note that in any innovation, there will always be a small group of individuals who never adopt the innovation. Knowing that the tipping point is around 15 percent of users, would it not be easiest to seek out the other innovators and early adopters to champion your cause? Between the two, you will hit the point of no return. It will take a lot less energy and frustration to then try to convince an early majority or especially a laggard to change into an innovator or early adopter!

Innovation and Communication

This example of innovation dates to 2015, when I was a chief nursing officer, and was novel and progressive at that time. We had what is now the very typical problem of throughput challenges, moving our patients out of the emergency department and into medical/surgical and critical care beds and at the same time the problem of expediting discharged patients. We used what is now described as a human-centered design process and pulled together some of the nurse leaders, house supervisors, a couple of physicians, and a few charge nurses to explore options of what would help us to improve this problem.

Our problem was a lack of communication of pending missions and discharges, as well as the issue of who was an observation patient so they could be managed appropriately. Remember, we did everything via pen and paper, and if you were sophisticated, you would incorporate spreadsheets. Software that solved these types of problems was still relatively new, and cloud-based services did not yet exist. At that time, there were not many throughput-related solutions on the market, and we explored a couple of platforms and identified a specific vendor to track patients through the hospital journey.

We reconvened our group to create process rules regarding topics such as the timeliness of entering pending discharges and admissions and the accuracy of identifying observation patients so the appropriate staff and physicians were aware and could proceed accordingly with their care plans.

While the solution was a paradigm shift for all, we quickly learned through the unit-based staff and physicians that if we could more broadly communicate this information, it would be even more helpful so that everyone knew what was occurring on the unit. So, the second stage of our solution was to amplify this information, and in accordance with Health Insurance Portability and Accountability Act requirements, we placed a large flat-panel monitor screen in a location where the care team, unit clerks, physicians, nurses, food services, and environmental service could visualize. This meant that for the first time, staff and physicians knew how many pending discharges and admissions were intended for their unit. This helped everyone on the team to plan their day and improved communication across all disciplines.

To continue this innovative thinking, we took this a step further, and because the house supervisors were so integral to the throughput process, we identified the third stage of the solution and provided them with a tablet to make them mobile, which was not a common practice at that time. The house supervisors worked off paper tools, the notorious "clipboard," and had to frequently

(continued)

EXPERIENCE FROM THE FIELD (CONTINUED)

run back to the house supervisor office to update their computers for bed placement as well as to check on staffing. So, we took the next step of deploying tablets to allow the house supervisors to be mobile and see tracker screens without having to sit in their office.

The fourth and final step in this process was that the house supervisors explained that if we could place the staffing and scheduling software on their tablets, they could be out of their offices most of the time. So, we did this as well, which allowed them to manage staffing (resources) and patients (demands) across the hospital. While not a perfect system, this was transformative and improved patient care, staff satisfaction, throughput, and staffing.

Bonnie Clipper, DNP, MA, MBA, RN, CENP, FACHE, FAAN
Founder & CEO, Innovation Advantage

EXPERIENCE FROM THE FIELD

Professional Development and Organization Type

The structure of a professional development department in a system can be a challenge. What do you centralize at the system level and what do you do locally? The first step to get clarity as you make these decisions is to align with the goals of the system. Do they want to function as a holding company in which the system oversees individual business or as an operating company that values standardization as a means to efficiencies and cost containment? Think of your favorite fast-food restaurant when you think of an operating company with standardization and efficiencies. When you order a sandwich and fries, do you expect to receive the same meal in Seattle as you do in Baltimore?

Once the question of function is answered, you can determine how much structure and processes to maintain centrally. If you find you are functioning as an operating company, more will be centralized than decentralized. It makes sense that if all processes are the same, there are efficiencies gained by one teaching many and driving to the same goals. If, however, you are functioning as a holding company, there may be too many nuances to be efficient in teaching anything centrally. Regardless of the philosophy, the resources need to be allocated in order to function as a professional practice department and have the same outcomes in each facility.

Deborah Maust Martin, DNP, RN, NE-BC, FACHE, Colibri Group, St. Louis, MO

Creativity without Stifling

An important step in creating standardization is to have a common language and set of definitions. I also believe that having a policy on policies is a must. This is where the common language and the common processes for standardization are noted for the organization where everyone has access to it. Communication and collaboration are also important components in creativity. We will discuss this

---

EXPERIENCE FROM THE FIELD

Innovation through Courage, Credibility, and Collaboration

Creativity and thinking outside the box to generate new ideas is important. But putting these ideas into action in complex systems is greatly dependent on your courage, credibility, and ability to collaborate. It takes courage to call out a problem or opportunity, identify a potential solution, address a sacred cow, or expose a deviant practice, all while risking missteps and failures. And it takes personal credibility to gain the confidence of others so that they are willing to collaborate and come along beside you, investing their time, energy, and resources.

Here are a few tips to strengthen your courage and credibility before jumping into an innovation project:

- Establish yourself as someone others can trust. Be that person others can count on, delivering on your promises (aka—TRUST = INFLUENCE).

- Show your manager or supervisor your potential in your work. Deliver quality in your everyday activities. Complete projects on time. Come to meetings prepared. Be a student of "best practices."

- Build your relationships! Get to know people throughout the organization, people with diverse views, skills, and roles. Be thoughtful and courteous. Genuinely give credit to others for their contributions.

- Learn to clearly define a problem or opportunity. Use clear descriptions, metrics, pictures, diagrams, and so on. Avoid vagaries and words such as "always" and "never."

- When you bring up a problem, include a thoughtful solution or next step toward resolving the issue.

- Get more comfortable with trying new things and the messiness of learning. Get familiar with taking two steps forward, one step back, as you intentionally try new things and find yourself back in a novice role.

Through consistency with these activities, you will grow your courage, influence, and credibility as a problem solver and innovator who can be trusted.

Exemplar to follow "Creativity without Stifling"
By Kathy A. Scott, PhD, RN, FACHE
and Bridget Sarikas
Partners and Co-Founders, L3 Fusion LLC

more in chapter 9, but start thinking about those components now. How can you be innovative and standardized?

We discussed the importance of innovation and standardization in this chapter, but it must be done through collaboration. No one person has all the right answers, and by working together, looking at the literature, and making it a priority to place the best evidence into practice, there is still so much room to be innovative. What can you do to be innovative even with the best evidence?

Key Points

- Quite often the issue of innovation and standardization is change.

- An innovation is merely a good idea until it is diffused.

- In order to make innovation happen, the whole world does not have to adopt it at the same time!

- Standardization allows health care providers to provide equality in care.

- Standardizing policies, procedures, and other such documents is no easy task.

CHAPTER 5

Facilitating and Managing Change

A long habit of not thinking a thing wrong gives
it the superficial appearance of being right.

—Thomas Paine

One of the most difficult and often painful processes in any organization or system is change. Either you hear people complain about too much change or that change is happening too slowly. Either way, all people complain about change at some point. To innovate and operationalize standardization, change must occur using change agents, theories, leadership skills, frontline staff, and management. Each organization is part of some system, and a system consists of more than one organization, so change within a system is dependent upon each organization's success. Remember in chapter 4 to consider negative and positive feedback loops as you read about change. This chapter is about change, the components of change that organizations need to consider and how to facilitate change so that everyone in an organization is successful.

Change and Organizations: Processes and Theories

Most of us understand *change* as any dictionary would define it: the act, process, or result of becoming or being made different; an alteration, a substitution, even a transformation. As nurse leaders, we are here to do just that: lead in the system to make those changes that transform our profession and health care system. Change is not simple, partly because it involves people. It has been estimated that up to 67 percent of well-formulated strategies fail due to poor execution (Carucci, 2017). To be successful in change or transformation, we all must recognize the roles we play in supporting or not supporting change. If we continue to have the same (although once successful) responses to new challenges, the change will inevitably suffer a decline and eventual failure (Kanter, 2009). Our health care delivery system faces just such a challenge, and unfortunately, we have been responding with old strategies (Haddon, 1989, p. 151).

Jim Collins's (2001) premise in *Good to Great* is that the primary indicator of great companies is a focus on not only the strategic goals to be accomplished but also the avoidance or cessation of counterproductive activities. How many sacred cows do we have in nursing? How many processes do we insist on doing ourselves because we think no one else could possibly do them? The organization needs to manage, avoid, and decrease organizational- and system-level counterproductive activities, and so do nurses at the unit and individual levels. Current methods for prioritizing and rolling out change initiatives need to be updated to include an account of business goals and employee capacity, which includes cessation strategies (Safar et al., 2007; Voelpel et al., 2004).

Change Agents

Change agents are usually the people called early adopters in the diffusion of innovation adopter curve (see table 4.1). An innovation starts slow, but through the change agents who actively diffuse the innovation, it will pick up speed as more people adopt it. Note that change agents are usually different from the innovator. Innovators are usually the leading-edge researcher, thinker, or inventor. These individuals might be labeled as eccentric by others. The change agent can be considered the idea broker for the innovator. The change agent is the promoter of new ideas, solutions, and directions. They read the research and see the use in the innovation, then translate the research.

Change Theories

There are multiple change theories, and quite often, "the" change theory used by an organization turns more into a buzzword. Unfortunately, many talk about change theories, but few understand them. And fewer understand the inherent risk in using them. However, change theories are widely used in most organizations, so it is advisable to try to understand how these theories can contribute to successful change. I will discuss three change theories next, but there are many more.

As touched on in the last chapter, Roger's diffusion of innovation is also considered a change theory but usually used in concert with others. You may also hear colleagues talking about Six Sigma and Lean. These are also very important and used within the change process and theory. Both are additive in that they are management practices to improve effectiveness and efficiencies and decrease waste and error. Within process improvement, you will expect to hear any and all of these terms, theories, and management processes in use.

Lewin's three-step change theory
For many nurses, this may be the most familiar change theory. Often this one is used as an example in nursing texts in the context of health education and promotion for patients. This change theory was developed by Kurt Lewin, a pioneer in group and organizational psychology, who noted that the three steps to change are

1. Unfreezing

2. Change

3. Refreezing (Hussain et al., 2018)

Unfreezing is the process of changing behavior and overcoming the strains of individual resistance and group conformity. It can also motivate participants by preparing them for change, building trust and recognition of the need for change, and having them actively participate in recognizing problems and brainstorming solutions within a group (Hussain et al., 2018). There are three potentials ways to unfreeze:

- Increase the driving forces that direct behavior away from the existing situation or status quo

- Decrease the restraining forces that negatively affect the movement from the existing equilibrium

- A combination of the two methods listed above

For instance, let us look at this from the perspective of helping an individual to stop smoking. To help them unfreeze, you will need to help the individual realize the pros and cons of quitting smoking, understand that there are more pros to quitting, and get them motivated to change. Unless a person is self-motivated to change, it will not happen.

In the second phase of change—*change* itself—an individual, a group, or an entire organization needs to move the target system to a new level of equilibrium. Three potential actions can assist in the movement:

- Persuading employees to agree that the status quo is not beneficial to them and encouraging them to view the problem from a fresh perspective

- Working together on a quest for new, relevant information

- Connecting the views of the group to well-respected, powerful leaders who also support the change (Kritsonis, 2005)

In the second phase, it is important to get the input from those who do the work! Change is a process, not an event. If they are a part of the problem solving, they will have an easier time with this change. Also, it is important to share the new vision with everyone. If an individual knows the direction in which they are headed or the desired outcome, they are much more likely to buy into the work that needs to be done to accomplish the change. Additionally, provide time for individuals to figure out their role in the new process.

The last step is *refreezing*, where we seek to stabilize the new equilibrium resulting from the change by balancing both the driving and restraining forces. The change has been accepted, and now you need to stabilize it and make it (for the moment) constant. One action that can be used to implement Lewin's third step in nursing organizations is to reinforce new patterns and institutionalize them through formal and informal mechanisms, including policies, procedures, standards of care, care pathways, and other mechanisms used widely by all employees.

Many of us do not want to unfreeze again for a long time! The process of any given change might be long, problematic, or intense. Think about the last time you were involved in a change: you probably went through some similar steps and were thankful when it was done! But what would you think if an innovation or new evidence suggested the need to change again? Would you jump up to make the change, or would you even want to know? We often make change so difficult (and there are so many changes that are always occurring) that we do not revisit change in a timely manner or even look to see if the outcomes are what we anticipated. So, while a policy or procedure may be the right way to freeze a change, if you really do not need one, do not create one.

Lippitt's change theory
Elaborating on Lewin's three-step change theory, social scientists Ronald Lippitt, Jeanne Watson, and Bruce Westley (1958) created a seven-step theory that focuses more on the role and responsibility of the change agent than on the evolution of the change. Remember, the change agent is the person who really drives the innovation into everyday practice. This is a pivotal role, and sustained change cannot exist without someone acting in this role. To be successful, the change agent needs to follow the following seven steps:

1. Diagnose the problem.

2. Assess the motivation and capacity for change.

3. Assess the resources and motivation of the change agent. This includes the change agent's commitment to change, power, and stamina.

4. Choose progressive change objects. In this step, action plans are developed and strategies are established.

5. Define the roles of the change agents so that expectations are clear. Examples of roles are cheerleader, facilitator, and expert.

6. Maintain the change. Communication, feedback, and group coordination are essential elements in this step of the change process.

7. Gradually terminate from the helping relationship. The change agent should gradually withdraw from their role over time. This will occur when the change becomes part of the organizational culture (Lippitt et al., 1958, pp. 58–59).

Their model and findings note that changes are more likely to be stable if they spread to neighboring systems or to subparts of the system immediately affected (Kritsonis, 2005). Quite often, organizations may have a unit or a system that has just one organization pilot a change. Using this method, the lessons learned and the support for isolated change can become lost and limit the success of the rollout of this innovation to other units or organizations. Other units or organizations may have nuances not considered in the pilot, and the time and attention needed to successfully modify and roll out an innovation may not be given to subsequent post pilot units or organizations. There is so much change, and we move quickly to the next problem. So a new initiative may take priority and focus away and not allow for a fuller focus to ensure successful change in the remaining neighboring systems. An innovative idea is not truly an innovation until it moves to the early adopters.

The great piece of this theory: noting the important role of the change agent. This role cannot be underplayed or undervalued. As a nurse leader, you might know your role as the change agent, or maybe you have been the change agent and never realized it. It is important to understand that this role is pivotal. The change agent is not the lifelong champion of a change. As the change agent, you should focus on embedding the change so well that you are out of a job.

Prochaska and DiClemente's change theory
The original purpose of the Prochaska and DiClemente (1984) model of change behavior was to be used by health care professionals to understand a patient's process for changing certain health behaviors. Since this model has been extended to areas outside of health care, the model defines a more general process of change and therefore tends to be less specific (Kritsonis, 2005). Prochaska and DiClemente found that people pass through a series of stages when change occurs: precontemplation, contemplation, preparation, action, and maintenance. The progression, and therefore the model, is cyclical, not linear, as individuals may go back and forth between stages as they progress in change, sometimes stepping "backward." Quite often, this theory is used to explain the process used by individuals as they stop smoking as well. The five steps and their definitions are as follows:

1. *Precontemplation:* An individual is unaware or fails to acknowledge the problems and does not engage in any change process activities.

2. *Contemplation:* The individual raises consciousness of the issue and begins to think about changing their behavior.

3. *Preparation:* When the individual is ready to change their behavior and plans to do so within the next two weeks.

4. *Action:* An increase in coping with behavioral change when the individual begins to engage in change activities.

5. *Maintenance:* Reinforcing the change to establish the new behavioral change to the individual's lifestyle and norms (Kritsonis, 2005, pp. 4–5).

These stages may last anywhere from six months up to the life span of the individual or organization. This is a very detailed process and very applicable to a person making lifestyle changes. However, different types of change, maybe a clinical practice change or a scheduling change, may require a different change process, one that fits the change that you wish to make. Think through your change, and decide which process seems right and own it.

GE Change Acceleration Process (CAP)

In 2006, General Electric (GE) launched its Leadership, Innovation, and Growth (LIG) program, created to weave innovation and growth into every aspect of their businesses, not just having managers reexamine their capabilities, processes, metrics, organizational structures, and deployment of resources. Through a specialized education program, GE created a process for change that led leaders to reconsider how they individually and collectively led: their behavior, their roles, and how they spent their time (Prokesch, 2009). In that program, they created and defined the GE Change Acceleration Process (CAP) as the process of moving the current state of the process/service/product to an improved state by catalyzing (speeding up) the transition state (Six Sigma, 2023).

The seven steps to the CAP are as follows:

• Leading change

• Creating a shared need

• Shaping a vision

• Mobilizing commitment

• Making change last

• Monitoring progress

• Changing systems and structures (Von Der Linn, 2009)

Projects fail for a variety of reasons, but critically important is ensuring the infrastructure is aligned with the objectives (Dawson, 2020). So, for managers to lead change, they need to balance the steps such as creating a shared need, with managing the present while creating the future. While managing change, it is also important to consider the following components in addition to the steps.

- *Team training:* Managers have an opportunity to reach consensus on the barriers to change.

- *Hard versus soft barriers:* Consider both the hard barriers to change (organizational structure, capabilities, and resources) and the soft barriers (how the members of the leadership team individually and collectively behave and spend their time).

- *Short term versus long term:* Simultaneously managing the present and creating the future.

- *Common vocabulary:* Beyond providing new concepts that would make people look at their businesses and themselves differently, the course created a common vocabulary of change (Prokesch, 2009).

These components can be applied as design principles for any change management program, not just a program concerning growth. The program's aim was to embed growth into the DNA of GE. Basically, they were creating and educating teams to lead the businesses to think about organic growth day in and day out—to be constantly on the lookout for opportunities and to create inspirational strategic visions that would enlist their troops in the cause. GE took this beyond the individual to a team approach to making change occur. Keep in mind that this is a change process and should not be considered a management structure. Additionally, this does have bureaucratic undertones that could benefit from radical management structure.

A Personal Note about Change Theories

The biggest issue with change theories is that you really need to connect an innovation piece from each of them to apply it specifically to your organization! Once you have refrozen the change or modified a behavior, individuals and organizations think they are done with that task and do not have to worry about it ever again! Like I have mentioned before, we cannot forget about the negative and positive feedback loops.

There is a reason why we should ensure that our nursing organizations have review policies and procedures at a specific and timely frequency: all the new knowledge generated! We create structures that are so frozen and bureaucratic that they fumble with being fluid and open to change, even though we know that any change refrozen should not stay frozen without being revisited frequently!

Most important, do not freeze things so well that it takes a lot of effort to unfreeze them. That sounds counterintuitive to standardization, but a balance must be maintained between innovation and standardization. As Margaret Wheatley (2006) noted, an open system needs to be taking input from the environment and responding appropriately to feedback.

Shared Leadership and Bureaucracy

In the beginning, health care was a mission: a mission of nuns, religious organizations, nurses, and physicians. Now that health care has moved under heavy federal regulation to provide a certain level of protection to patients, it really has become a type of inalienable right for us. The government's role in health care delivery occurred with the start of Social Security and increased with the initial Medicare creation. These changes occurred due to public demand for these services.

With all these changes at the national level came changes at the organizational level. Hospitals were asked to do more with less, which is now a recurring theme in our health care delivery system. Fifty years ago, a hospital's management structure was much simpler, with an administrator and a director of nursing and the necessary staff to provide patient care, housekeeping, and meals. Since then, with all the additional federal and state government regulations, hospitals and other health care organizations have had to quickly add staff: staff to manage quality, regulations, and finances. This was really the start of bureaucracy in health care organizations (Haddon, 1989, p. 151).

When the population grew, the science around health and our abilities to care and heal patients quickly grew too. Hospitals grew larger so that they could provide more services and be more productive and efficient. Becoming larger may make one more efficient in one aspect, but it does add complexity. Administrators then added even more complex structures and processes, as well as more staff, to manage this complexity. This created a large middle management level that slows the decision-making process down so much that organizations are increasingly incapable of adapting to change (Drucker, 1986).

Health care organizations continue on the same seemingly unbreakable cycle: external pressure from government ➔ increased internal complexity ➔ increased administrative staff ➔ increased alienation of staff ➔ increase pressure for more external change (Haddon, 1989, p. 151).

Exemplar: Leadership Reset in the Postpandemic World

In dynamic times such as these, organizations are pushed to act faster and perform with more flexibility and efficiency. This requires leadership at all levels of the organization. Hierarchical, top-down approaches are not adequate for today's many and ongoing challenges. Approaches are needed that allow for an effective response to the changes that enables organizational regeneration.

Surveys of the global and US workplace over the past several years have put a spotlight on the frustration of employees related to lack of clarity about their organization's processes for planning, organizing, and prioritizing workloads and tasks. In fact, it is estimated that the US workforce spends 60 percent of their time in mundane, time-consuming work rather than on their focused areas of expertise and skill—resulting in wasteful hours spent on duplicative and unnecessary work. This is the antithesis of meaningful work.

It is time for a **LEADERSHIP RESET.** This was needed before the pandemic but is even more important now. As leaders of change initiatives, it is important to gain insight into the organizational dynamics and context in which this change is to be implemented. This understanding comes through connection with the team in meaningful ways.

When leaders become better informed through connecting with their team in meaningful ways, amazing things can happen. We use a variety of forums to gain a better understanding of the following:

1) The new demands on the employees and team members—determine if demands need to be reduced, scope changed or clarified, priorities reevaluated, and/or processes retooled.

2) How much control the team members want and need to be able to do their best work and stay engaged with the organization—determine what controls are too tight and what controls need to be strengthened.

3) Whether the team members have adequate support to get the needed results—determine if they have adequate resources to get the job done in the expected timeframe. Ascertain if there is enough slack in the system to allow for adequate problem solving and learning. Ask the team if there are new and different ways you can provide the needed support.

The work of leaders moving forward is to build strong teams that willingly choose to contribute their strengths, passions, and talents to the greater good. This requires a leadership mindset that genuinely respects the team members and trusts in their capacity to be generous, contributing, and kind. And it also requires new structures for communication, problem solving, and decision-making that capitalize on the talents of the team.

Kathy Scott, PhD, RN, FACHE and Bridget Sarikas

Patient and Staff Experience Transformation in an Obstetrics Unit

A few years ago, a new director joined a labor and delivery team in a small suburban hospital in Arizona. The team was struggling to find their way after a string of less than desirable patient outcomes and community perceptions that matched those outcomes. After taking time to get to know the team and processes, several opportunities became known. There was a focus on team and a lack of focus on purpose. Practices were built with a large dependence on individual knowledge and skill. There was a lack of systematic processes and guardrails. The team had extreme ownership and pride and therefore felt solely responsible for system breakdown resulting in the poor outcomes. Patient experience was also inconsistent, with some patients loving the care they received and others feeling like just another number. The team was burnt out from holding it all together. Staff felt unsupported and appeared jealous that the organization's focus was on patient satisfaction. It was no shock that their employee engagement and satisfaction was low, and the only positive from the survey was they liked working with each other.

Shifting to a patient- and family-centered environment was going to take a 180-degree change in mind-set. Change had to start from within. As their leader, the job ahead was to connect the hearts of the caregivers to the work and show them how they made a difference and could improve the quality and feeling of care in their practice. This included posting score cards of key metrics in the breakroom and transparently sharing all patient experience data, including all comments. Positive comments were left unblinded, and the negative comments had names of caregivers blinded. Staff who were called out in a positive way had their comments read aloud in the staff meeting and given notes with small treats from their leader. Those mentioned in negative comments were met with in private to share the comments and talk through what they remembered about the encounter, with time for self-reflection and coaching to improve interactions. All were treated as learning opportunities through mentoring and coaching, without punishment. Unit leaders rounded on every patient and family in the unit to hear their experience and what could be done better. Those rounds also included pointed questions about areas that were eliciting lower survey scores and feedback to see what insights could be gained in real time and make corrections. One such question was, "On our recent surveys, we have seen our 'room kept clean' scores lower than we would like them to be. Is there anything that you have encountered during your stay that we could do a better job of cleaning?" During these rounds, the leaders also asked if there were any staff who stood out to the patients. They would then immediately

(continued)

share that feedback directly with the team member. Staff were empowered to do their own real-time rounding and service recovery in the moment to make each patient and family's experience superb. Patients who shared opportunities through their comments on the Hospital Consumer Assessment of Healthcare Providers and Systems HCAHP surveys were contacted to learn more fully of the experience. The insights from these experiences were shared with the team at the staff meetings to bring the patients to life. The staff were given the opportunity to share their stories of rounding and service recovery. The team adopted the motto, "Don't be the one!" To them this meant, do not be the one called out in a patient's experience that made something not good when the rest of the team worked really hard to make it great.

Adding tools to the patient- and family-centered tool box for the staff was meant to empower and support them in making the patient experience remarkable. Birth plan templates given to families when they took their Labor and Delivery tour and whiteboards in the patient rooms that called out the most important part of the patient's labor and then postpartum plan helped the team know what to focus on. Learning the patient's significant other or support person's name as well as the planned name for the baby also helped to personalize the experience for each family and bring staff and patients closer together.

Within a year, the team had moved over 15 points in the percentile rankings. By 18 months, they were leading the health system OB units in patient experience. The extreme ownership they originally espoused was still there, but now the team safeguarded the patient's care and experience. The team beamed with pride as other units around the system reached out to learn about their "secret sauce" and how to start a wave of transformation of their own.

Amy Yates, MSN, RN, CENP

Does this sound familiar? The interesting point is that this was discussed in 1989—and it is still true today. This cycle can only be broken with change, internal change that is planned and chosen with staff input (Haddon, 1989, p. 151). Sounds like the radical management we discussed in chapter 2! That is because one of those key components in radical management is shared leadership.

Shared leadership is not and should not be considered another layer or another level of bureaucracy but rather the correct process by which internal processes manage external pressures. Shared leadership goes by many names, including shared governance and dynamic governance. Shared leadership is considered a structure by which professionals can practice their autonomous professional decision-making abilities. Sharing decisions allows more decisions to be made and changes to be implemented more quickly and more efficiently if done correctly. Shared leadership is also known as shared governance and is similar to dynamic governance.

Lasting and Meaningful Change

Once an organization or system has implemented the change, it is absolutely necessary to ensure that it does not become unraveled when the focus is on the next new project. First, make sure that the change is needed. I know we just went

---

EXPERIENCE FROM THE FIELD

Successful Change

Great ideas and best practices are commonplace in a highly functioning organization, yet multiple processes can result in various outcomes, confusion, and unpredictability. Systems that are highly organized and use a solid infrastructure have in place a method of approaching work that is effective, although not always efficient. The effectiveness comes from project management, which helps move a group of diverse and talented experts in a direction that achieves results. This is the easy part. As a facility leader, I have learned that the rollout of new structures and processes is where the rubber meets the road. Implementing in small, medium, and large facilities can be quite different, and there needs to be a distinction between what is negotiable and nonnegotiable in the process steps. Achieving the clinical or operational outcome must remain the overall goal. Clear communication in a culture of trust is essential for a system to safely and effectively implement across diverse facilities. Tweaks to the process, made with solid rationale and information, are essential in achieving results across a system.

One common challenge for me working in systems is the balance required in representing the facility and the system simultaneously. I often said to my team that our job was to "have one foot in the system and one foot in the facility at all times." It was often difficult to effectively communicate the rationale of system approaches and changes to a group that was already doing quite well as it was. The system wants the whole organization to change, even if parts of the organization are doing well. My role as a clinical leader required that I use information, data, and integrity in communicating facility and system needs so that change could occur safely and effectively. This is not easy and is sometimes perceived as normal pushback against change. What is the difference? This is what leadership is about in a system—knowing the difference and representing "the right thing" for the sake of safe and excellent patient care.

Colleen Hallberg, RN, MSN

---

over innovation and keeping up with best practice, but often change may be a pet project that is not based in evidence or will not make a positive impact on staff or patient outcomes.

Once you know the change is needed, make sure that you are knowledgeable in change theories, use a change theory to guide you, ensure a shared vision for the change (shared leadership is a great way to do that), have a change agent, monitor progress, and embed the change into everything applicable. Focus on not making the change tedious, and do not let it take over everything that you and others do. The worst thing you can do is cause change fatigue in yourself and others.

Change is a complex process. As a nurse leader, you will be involved with change, whether it affects what you do or you are making the change that affects others. Remember, if you do not like change, you will like irrelevance even less.

Key Points

- Health care organizations have been created more from effect than cause and are reactive still instead of proactive.

- The definition of change is the act, process, or result of changing, as an alteration or transformation.

- Change agents are a must as they are the ones who actively work on diffusing the innovation.

- Organizational bandwidth refers to the number of competing priorities that an organization is working on or can work on successfully at any given time.

- Shared leadership is considered a structure by which professionals can practice their autonomous professional decision-making abilities.

CHAPTER 6
All Nurses Are Leaders

One of the hardest tasks of leadership is
understanding that you are not what you are,
but what you're perceived to be by others.

—Edward L. Flom, CEO of Florida Steel

One of the most valuable pieces of knowledge I have about leadership is that the type of relationships you have with others is of utmost importance. As noted by Edward Flom, an important aspect of leadership is not just knowing who you are but how you are perceived. You get that input through many avenues, but the most beneficial way, the one way that is not destructive, is though relationships. Good ones. How many times have you received feedback on your work as a leader or as a person that was less than flattering?

Maybe something occurred and the end result was not the view of yourself that you wanted people to remember? Having good relationships with people opens the doors for upfront and honest feedback so that you can become a better person, a better nurse, and a better leader. And when something less than becoming does occur (it will), then you will more likely be granted grace.

The key thing to remember as a person who happens to be a nurse is that you are a leader regardless of your position, regardless of whether or not you wanted to be a leader. You are a nurse. You are a leader. Leaders do not have to be managers to lead. And sometimes a manager does not act like a leader. The American Nurses

Association (ANA) Social Policy Statement speaks to the commitment and accountability you have as a professional nurse:

> Nurses as members of a knowledge-based health profession and as licensed healthcare professionals, must answer to patients, nursing employers, the board of nursing, and the civil and criminal court system when the quality of patient care provided is compromised or when allegations of unprofessional, unethical, illegal, unacceptable or inappropriate nursing conduct, actions, or responses arise. (ANA, 2010)

We are here to serve our patients, our community, and our profession. Being a leader is a great responsibility. Too often nurses think of a nurse leader as someone in a management role or someone with a management title. As nurses, we place a hierarchy to our management roles, believing that a chief nursing officer or executive is the pinnacle of nursing leadership. People often confuse management and leadership when they are not the same.

Too often we are so concerned with our own worlds that we do not see all the opportunities right outside our boxes, right outside our comfort zones. A manager who is a leader will listen to their staff. Often, the staff do have all the answers, and that may make a manager uncomfortable, but it will not make a leader uncomfortable. Leaders know they do not hold all the answers. Leaders are there to remove barriers and open the way for their staff to do what they do best: providing excellent patient care.

This chapter discusses the nurse as a leader, as an individual, and within various professional roles. Read each section to understand what others might be going through in their leadership roles and what others have learned, and take from it what you can to continue your growth as a leader—whatever role that may be. This is not about hierarchy but about different but equal roles in leadership.

Leadership Traits

There are many definitions of a leader and certainly many leadership traits that are valued by nurses, health care professionals, and others. Quite often in nursing, we tend to stick to nursing literature to define and understand concepts. It is good practice to know what is valued in nursing and to know what is going on in other industries as well. Borrowing terms, concepts, and thoughts from other disciplines will make our own discipline stronger and keep us from rebuilding the same wheel!

In this section, I will review valued nursing leadership traits as well as leader traits from other industries.

Transformational Leadership

In nursing, we value transformational leadership as an ideal leadership type. Transformational leadership is one of the five American Nurses Credentialing Center (ANCC) Magnet Recognition Model components. But what is transformational leadership, and how does one become transformational?

Good questions!

Transformational leadership is a theory that was developed by James McGregor Burns in 1978. The theory was developed to further address the aspects of an organization that lead to success, encourage enthusiasm among an organization's employees, and identify the values employees place on their work (Burns, 1978).

The transformational leadership style allows for the recognition of areas in which change is needed and guides change by inspiring followers and creating a sense of commitment (Smith, 2011), not by telling people what to do and how to do it. Burns further notes that good performance from employees comes from rewarding compliance (transactional) or motivating to meet higher-order needs (transformational). Transformational leaders have been associated with better outcomes in nursing, which include

- Improving job satisfaction

- Empowering nurses

- Strengthening organizational commitment and increasing productivity

- Reducing turnover and increasing retention

- Enhancing work group collaboration

- Improving patient outcomes (Boamah et al., 2018; Wong et al., 2013)

Further work on transformational leadership has been done by Kouzes and Posner (2000) through the model of exemplary leadership practice. They note that leadership is not about personality; it is about behavior, which has an observable set of skills and abilities. There are five characteristics that exemplary leaders demonstrate and behaviors in which they engage:

- Challenge the process

- Inspire a shared vision

- Enable others to act

- Model the way

- Encourage the heart (Kouzes & Posner, 2000)

An instrument to measure these concepts, called the Leadership Practices Inventory (LPI), has been used in nursing to assess both the effectiveness of managers as leaders and the levels of commitment, engagement, and satisfaction in those who follow. Researchers have found that transformational leadership is a universally accepted and preferred leadership style, with increased levels of satisfaction under this style (Caza et al., 2021).

The transformational leadership style inspires others to develop and implement effective leadership characteristics. The goal of transformational leadership is for the leader and the follower to discover meaning and purpose in relation to their work, in addition to growth and maturity. Are there situations in which a transformational leadership style may not be the best approach? Possibly. But I would encourage leaders and managers to lead through transformation, be cognizant of when and where they slip into other leadership styles, and incorporate reflective practices.

As a nurse leader, you may not have a manager role where you have followers based on reporting structure. But as a leader, you may have followers in other nurses who have found you to be someone who has shown them how to find meaning and purpose in their own work. As a nurse, you play an instrumental role in the culture of your work environment. You either co-create a good working environment or contribute to a negative one. What type of leader will you be as part of your work environment?

Leadership in Other Industries

It is important to always look beyond our own discipline and industry to know what others are doing that can be of use to our profession. While the LPI is used across many industries, not just nursing or health care, it is something that is most widely acknowledged and used within nursing.

Going outside of nursing gives us a chance to understand the issues facing others in leadership and the knowledge they may have used to address those issues.

A good example is General Electric again. Researchers and organizations alike strive to define and teach the next set of leadership skills needed for the future. Here, GE has developed a set of individual growth values (table 6.1).

GE is known for its leadership university and the change processes that they have developed over decades of work. This work was originally intended for employees and teams internally, but many outside of GE have had the fortune of experiencing this education. In addition to the individual leader, it is recognized that having successful teams is an important part of leadership, as much as personal leadership. The growth values GE believes are necessary for innovating are taught in their team leadership program (Prokesch, 2009). In nursing and health care, we have worked in teams for decades.

With the move to value-based care, the focus on the care continuum, and the development of new innovative care models for the future, leadership in teams, especially transdisciplinary teams, will be vital regardless of the setting or your role!

How can you use these growth values in your role on a team (maybe one with shared leadership) to make the difference in patient care? Think about these values within a radical management context too!

In addition to the GE growth values, both the current and past CEOs of GE, Jack Welch and Jeff Immelt, have noted their own lists of valued leadership traits (Aykac, 2013). Even within the same organization, high-level organizational change occurs, and so does the evolution of leadership in the same organization. Jack Welch, former CEO of GE, was a leader over many decades. His philosophy, which

Table 6.1. GE Growth Values (Prokesch, 2009)

TRAIT	DEFINITION
Outward focus	Defines success through the customer's eyes. Is in tune with industry dynamics.
Thinking clearly	Seeks simple solutions to complex problems. Is decisive and focused. Communicates clear and consistent priorities.
Imagination	Generates new and creative ideas. Is resourceful and open to change. Takes risks on both people and ideas.
Inclusiveness	Is a collaborator. Respects others' ideas and contributions. Creates excitement, drives engagement, builds loyalty and commitment.
Showing expertise	Has in-depth domain knowledge and credibility built on experience. Continuously develops self.

influenced his understanding of leadership, was that leaders need to accept change and teach employees how important it is. Additionally, he believed that managing less is best and that employees will step up to accomplish great things if you give them room. Jack Welch noted five important traits of leadership:

- Ambition and energy

- Desire to lead

- Honesty and integrity

- Self-confidence

- Intelligence

The former CEO of GE, Jeff Immelt, notes that his success is due in part to 10 keys to leadership:

1. Understanding the breadth, depth, and context of your purpose and objective in the world

2. Simplifying on a continual basis

3. Aligning and managing time by mandating leader priorities

4. Measuring outcomes and rewarding employees accordingly

5. Setting a direction for the organization

6. Using communication to align people with that direction

7. Taking personal responsibility

8. Leaving a few things unsaid to allow employees to problem solve and execute to a greater organizational benefit

9. Liking people and treating them fairly

10. Mentoring and encouraging the completion of personal goals within the organization

While there may be several more lists of leadership traits and ideals from GE and other organizations, they are all similar in nature, and each leader recognized that they felt it was those traits that led to their success. There is a lot of research and suggestions about leadership traits, and many of these traits fall somewhere between a bureaucratic and a radical management style. How can you take these leadership traits and forge your own path?

While some of these traits may feel more appropriate for a formal leader in a management position, what trait can you use to grow yourself into making change and innovation occur?

NAM's The *Future of Nursing*

Starting in 2008, the Robert Wood Johnson Foundation (RWJF) and the Institute of Medicine (IOM, as it was named at the time) launched a two-year initiative in response to the need to assess and transform the nursing profession. The IOM appointed the Committee on the RWJF Initiative on the Future of Nursing with the purpose of producing a report that would make recommendations for an action-oriented blueprint for the future of nursing. Through its deliberations, the committee developed four key messages published in *The Future of Nursing: Leading Change, Advancing Health* report:

One Nurse's Leadership Style

Leading Outside Traditional Nurse Roles

I have to admit, being hired as the Executive Director of the Arizona Nurses Association had its leadership challenges. I was used to leading nurses as a hospital manager, leading patients as a Diabetes Educator, and leading students as nursing faculty. But none of my nurse training (or so I thought) prepared me to lead a state-level advocacy nonprofit organization representing the interests of over 80,000 nurses! So I had to create my own leadership blueprint. I found the experience both exhausting and invigorating! What I learned was that our training and experience as

nurses do prepare us to step out of the box and embrace any leadership challenge. My leadership pearls of wisdom during my 10-year executive director tenure were always to perform an environmental scan of your surroundings, be a good listener, embrace thinkers that are the opposite of you, and surround yourself with your own "kitchen cabinet," some close nurse colleagues who you can bounce ideas off in a safe environment. Finally, it is challenging to lead multiple projects and never encounter differences of opinion and conflict; therefore, consensus building is an important leadership attribute.

Robin Schaeffer, MSN, RN, CAE

- Nurses should practice to the full extent of their education and training.

- Nurses should achieve higher levels of education and training through an improved education system that promotes seamless academic progression.

- Nurses should be full partners, with physicians and other health care professionals, in redesigning health care in the United States.

- Effective workforce planning and policymaking require better data collection and information infrastructure (National Research Council [NRC], 2011, p. 4).

This report states that the US has the opportunity to transform its health care system and that nurses can and should play a fundamental role in this transformation. The power to improve the current regulatory, business, and organizational conditions does not rest solely with nurses; the government, businesses, health care organizations, professional associations, and the insurance industry all must play a role. But as nurses, as leaders, we all need to understand the basic system of regulations, businesses, and organizational conditions and work to change them. Working together, all of these diverse parties can lead and ensure that the health care system provides seamless, affordable, quality care that is accessible to all and leads to improved health outcomes (NRC, 2011).

A CONSIDERATION FOR SYSTEMS THINKING

A Reading Assignment

I strongly believe it is your professional responsibility to read or at least review both *The Future of Nursing: Leading Change, Advancing Health* report and *The Future of Nursing 2020–2030: Charting a Path to Achieve Health Equity*. There is a third report, published in 2016: *Assessing Progress on the Institute of Medicine Report The Future of Nursing*.

If you do not read the whole report, you must read the executive summary. I am surprised by the numbers of RNs and APRNs who not only have not read these reports but have not even heard of them. If you have not heard of these reports, you are not connected to your profession's organizations, at the state or national level. Being a leader includes an awareness of the major movements going on in your profession. The online PDF book versions of both are free! The first report is the second most downloaded report for the NAM.

You can go to the National Academy of Medicine (what use to be IOM) and search for both these reports: https://nam.edu/publications/.

The interesting thing about this report is that it took the NAM to tell nurses that we need to step up as leaders to make changes. Remember the earlier quote from Edward L. Flom about how leadership is about how others perceive you? The NAM perceives that we should be leaders. Our time is now; we need to step forward to fulfill expectations and lead our profession and health care system through the changes it needs. Each one of us.

The IOM report speaks to the future of nursing and what we need to do as nurses to lead the future. Other disciplines recognize our influence and abilities in the future of health care, but do we really? As a nurse, regardless of your position or role, ask yourself the following questions:

- How am I, as a nurse, influencing change?

- Am I slowing or blocking change or innovation, purposefully or accidentally?

- What am I afraid of losing in my role if change occurs?

- How do I define my role as an RN, and does that definition change if the future of nursing changes?

- Has that caused me to be a barrier in any way to change or even thinking innovatively?

Nurses can let others develop the roles of nursing for the future, or we can develop them for ourselves! If we are too busy blocking or slowing change, someone else will work around us and make change happen based on how they see the world. Change will happen. Change that affects us all, our current positions, our future positions, our profession. Digging our heels in will not stop it from happening, but it will stop our voices from being heard in the future.

Now, fast forward to the latest report from the NAM, *The Future of Nursing 2020–2030: Charting a Path to Achieve Health Equity*, published in 2021, which builds on the first report. This new report discusses where the nursing profession made advances, explains where we need to focus on for the future, and outlines vital next steps. The new report explores how nurses can work to reduce health disparities and promote equity while keeping costs at bay, utilizing technology, and maintaining patient- and family-focused care into 2030 (NASEM, 2021). Personally, as a nurse, I think only we can develop our future roles. But if we are not all involved in this, someone who is not a nurse will develop our roles for us. Do we want to fit into someone else's vision of the future or create our own? All of the information in this book is about informing your understanding of health care systems and the change you can make from whatever position you hold! It is your professional responsibility to be a leader.

Registered Nurses as Leaders

All RNs, regardless of position, are leaders. I have said that throughout the book, and I will continue to say it to the end. The moment you choose to be an RN, you choose to be a leader. As you read through this book, you might think, how does this all apply to me now? It all might not apply to you now, but take what does apply today and put it to use! Reexamine Jack Welch's traits of leadership:

1. Ambition and energy

2. Desire to lead

3. Honesty and integrity

4. Self-confidence

5. Intelligence

To improve your leadership abilities, ask yourself the following questions:

1. What trait do you admire the most?

2. What trait of a leader do you want to strengthen within yourself?

3. What one trait or behavior will you work on for your personal development this year?

4. Do you have a personal development plan at your organization in relationship to your yearly employee evaluation process that you can use to start developing your leadership abilities? If not, you can still create your own plan. (See the appendix for an example.)

You have read about many different leadership traits, some of which you are undoubtedly still thinking of how to apply to yourself! Only you are ultimately responsible for your own development, no one else. Do not wait for someone else to create a plan or talk to you about your own development. It may not happen.

Remember everything is related in a system, so it all applies to you—you just need to think it through! This is not about being a manager but a leader. But if you apply for a manager position, you might be asked about the strengths and weaknesses in your leadership traits. For instance, have you ever been on an interview panel for a new charge nurse or director as a clinical RN? Thinking through the list of transformational leadership traits, which behaviors or traits do you want in your manager? What questions can you ask of the candidate that will help you understand what type of leader they may be?

The First Follower: How to Create a Leader

Derek Sivers has a great TED video talk called "How to Start a Movement" (Sivers, 2010) and, as of early 2023, it has been viewed over 10 million times! Here, he points out that the first person to do something is not a leader until there is a first follower. Envision an outdoor concert. No one is dancing. Then, one person gets up and starts to dance. Here, he seems strange, and even though he was the first person, he is not a leader yet. But after a while, someone else gets up and starts to dance with him. Then more people get up to dance. This first person is the first follower. This first follower is the person who actually made the first person a "leader." There are a few important points to be gleaned from this video:

1. The first person is not a leader if no one follows; they are simply crazy.

2. The first follower is the one who creates a leader.

3. The leader had the wisdom to treat the first follower as an equal, which encouraged him to join and stay.

4. The people who come after everyone is already doing it are interesting, as they rush to get there when it is still cool but safe because a lot of people are doing it.

5. At some point, it may spread so far that people will risk ridicule for not joining.

6. Leaders are overrated; early (and especially first) followers provide an underrated form of leadership (Sivers, 2010).

This sounds like the diffusion of innovations. The innovator is the eccentric one, but the early adopters really make an idea an innovation. Then the rest adopt the innovation once it is safe.

We all know or remember a formal leader that no one followed or wanted to follow. They may have been our formal manager but we did not consider them a leader; we only followed them because we had to in our job. Yet someone had to be their first follower in order for them to have the leadership position. If we do not choose wisely who to follow, we might be that first follower, legitimizing the poor leadership qualities of the first person. Whether the first person is a good or bad leader, formal or informal, there is a role to play as the follower that sets up or destroys the legitimacy of that leader.

Advanced Practice Registered Nurses as Leaders

Everything that has been said so far in this chapter applies to APRNs, so there is no reason to repeat it. However, there are some unique differences for all APRNs to consider regarding their role as *Advanced Practice* RNs. The APRN Consensus Model for Regulation (2008 designates four APRN roles: Certified Nurse Practitioners (CNPs), Certified Nurse Midwives (CNMs), Clinical Nurse Specialists (CNSs), and Certified Registered Nurse Anesthetists (CRNAs).

These roles tend to differ from state to state; however, the consensus model has standardized the language and requirements around licensure, accreditation, certification, and education (better known as LACE) of APRNs. The goal is to pass legislation in each state and territory that reflects this standardization. This is an important step for APRNs to further their leadership in our health care systems. The *Future of Nursing* report states that all RNs need to practice to the full extent of their education and license. Practicing to the full extent is for both RNs and APRNs. Using each role to the full extent requires leadership to change state and federal barriers as well any local or facility-based barriers such as medical staff bylaws.

APRNs in all their roles are uniquely positioned to lead changes in our health care system across the care continuum. As per the APRN consensus model, all are able to provide care across the continuum and the system:

- CNPs provide care along the wellness–illness continuum through a dynamic process in any setting across the care continuum.

- The CNS's role is to integrate care across the continuum and through three spheres of influence: patient, nurse, and system.

- CNMs provide a full range of primary health care services to women throughout the life span, including gynecologic care, family planning services, preconception care, prenatal and postpartum care, childbirth, and care of the newborn across diverse settings, which may include home, hospital, birth center, and a variety of ambulatory care settings, including private offices and community and public health clinics.

- The CRNA is prepared to provide the full spectrum of patients' anesthesia care and anesthesia-related care for individuals across the life span in diverse settings, including hospital surgical suites and obstetrical delivery rooms, critical access hospitals, acute care, pain management centers, ambulatory surgical centers, and other outpatient settings (APRN Consensus Work Group, 2008).

Earlier in this chapter, I noted the first of the NAM *Future of Nursing* reports. While this report speaks to both RN and APRNs, pieces of this report have had a heavy influence already at a national level. In March 2014, the Federal Trade Commission staff issued a policy paper suggesting that state legislators should be cautious when evaluating proposals to limit the scope of practice of APRNs.

By limiting the range of services APRNs may provide and the extent to which they can practice independently, such proposals may reduce competition that benefits consumers, the paper states. If we are going to make change occur, then we need to take advantage of these statements and leverage them at every level in the system.

Keep in mind that the earliest study on the cost and effectiveness of nurse practitioners (NPs) was done in 1981 by the Office of Technology Assessment (OTA) and reported that NPs provided equivalent or improved medical care at a lower cost than physicians. This was the start of many studies showing the quality of care provided, yet as nurses, we are still fighting for an equal place in the system.

SOMETHING TO CONSIDER
If you want to see the extent of the fight against independent APRN practice, visit the American Medical Association website. They are quite clear and proud of their work to fight scope of practice expansion. What have you done to support the nursing profession, at both the RN and APRN level? Remember, silence is acquiescence.

CNS Standardization for Hospital Organizations

CNSs make valuable contributions to hospital organizations by improving quality for highly complex patient populations and enhancing professional nursing practice.

When the health care system is large and consists of multiple hospitals, standardization and cohesiveness among CNSs are essential.

Standardization can be accomplished in a number of ways and should always directly involve CNSs in facilitating and leading the decision-making process. Standardization of position descriptions, care delivery models, competencies, goal setting, orientation and credentialing, and reimbursement for certification/licensing requirements are examples of processes that should be considered for standardization. Frequent forums for sharing best practices and opportunities for sharing Evidence Based Practice (EBP) or research projects that have been presented at regional or national conferences should also be coordinated. Geographical barriers may present challenges to standardization; however, these challenges are possible to overcome, especially with advanced technology.

An example of an Advanced Practice Nurse (APN) project that will promote the advancement of CNS ideas, knowledge, and innovation into clinical practice is an APN subteam to develop the standardized CNS position description that will be implemented across the health organization. This can be accomplished face-to-face or through live meeting and a bridge line so all participants can view the documents simultaneously as they are being created and revised based on organizational needs, the CNS role, and the essential functions of the CNS role. This project can be expected to take three to six months or less to complete, depending on the frequency of meetings and the availability of the CNSs to attend the subteam meetings. As with any CNS system involvement, nursing management support is critical. The goal will be a product that reflects and captures the essence of the CNS role in any nursing specialty and will lead to job performance improvement.

This work can also be replicated for CNPs, CRNAs, and CNMs.

Position descriptions that are broad in scope can be adopted by CNSs in any specialty, especially if they can be individualized through addendums to address specific CNS role functions. Care delivery models can be utilized across specialties, as all CNSs work within the three spheres of influence: activities that support (1) patients/clients, (2) nurses, and (3) the hospital/organization. Competencies should be developed to ensure safe and ethical practices. Standardized orientation and credentialing processes are needed to ensure that newly hired CNSs are prepared to be successful in the APN role. Annual goal setting helps CNSs stay focused on priorities to help meet professional and organizational needs and enhance performance evaluation. It is highly recommended that reimbursement for certification and licensing requirements has parity with institutional policies for CNP reimbursement. Standardization of these priorities will contribute to the empowerment of CNSs and contribute to a continual spirit of inquiry that improves health care delivery.

Susan A. Phillips MSN, RN, PMHCNS-BC, PMHNP-BC

The NAM reports have brought a higher national level of attention to APRN practice issues, and the work of many professional associations has moved the needle farther in just the past few years. Making change takes leadership, which needs commitment and advocacy at national and grassroots levels. We know, based on decades of research, that APRNs are key in health care now and in the future as providers of health care services. As RNs and APRNs, we need to lead in the system and advance us all. Regardless of our role, we need to support and advance each other.

Nurse Leaders across Our Profession

There are many nurses who are not direct-care providers yet not in formal management positions either. These roles include nurse researchers, educators, case managers, care coordinators, quality specialists, and many more from all areas in health care. It is important to note once again that while we cannot go into every possible role a nurse may practice in, every nurse is a leader. These roles have unique barriers in demonstrating leadership. Here are some questions for you to ask yourself:

- How do you, in your role, assume leadership?

- How do you make change occur when you are neither at the point of care nor in a position of formal authority?

- How can you be a change leader?

- How do you lead working and partnering with others to facilitate change?

- How do you see change and innovation in your role and position?

- How do you lead your work with other direct-care RNs and APRNs?

As noted by Lesly Kelly, she was a leader in her role as a researcher. She ensured research findings were shared so that activities could be developed to increase wellness of nurses during the height of the COVID-19 pandemic. It is important that you know your role in change and innovation, as well as understand how you can make a difference in your role in leading in the system. Through this book, think about the impact you can make in the system, what impact you have already made in the system, and what your next steps in change are. We are all connected and a piece of a system. One of the keys is knowing as many of the moving internal and external parts as possible and collaborating with each other!

Nurse Managers and Executives as Leaders

This book is not exclusively about acute care nurses and leaders or leadership. So, I brought together multiple potential titles under one category. There are many things to consider about your role as a manager or executive in a system, whether you are new or experienced in your role.

New to a System

Even if you consider yourself an expert nurse, once you change roles or positions, you will find that you are not an expert any longer. You have a new organization, new people, new policies, procedures, and culture. And if you go into an organization thinking you are still the expert, you will quickly create relationship issues with your new coworkers who know more than you about the organization. You may be a content expert, but you need to recognize everything you do not know. It may be an uncomfortable feeling, but this is a great chance to show leadership skills! Great leaders admit they do not know everything.

It is important to have mentors and preceptors in a system to help you navigate the complexity. You certainly may feel overwhelmed in a new system: There are many dos and don'ts, as well as many people you need to "check with" who may "have oversight" on certain things outside of your own immediate context. It is different when you work in one building and not in a system. While it may be complex, if you are a visual learner, you will need to visualize a multilevel organizational chart. There are direct and matrix reporting relationships, and many times, new nurse leaders in a system are afraid to make change. A nurse leader who does not understand the complexity may have tried to make change and may have learned an unfortunate lesson from less-than-forgiving individuals.

It is important that you ask for a preceptor and seek a mentor who can help you navigate the politics of a complex multilevel organization. The worst thing a nurse manager can do is not lead. Your staff watches you and forms their opinions about their health care system through your ability to navigate successfully.

Being Experienced in a System

The experienced manger or executive should understand the culture, the processes, and the connectedness that are unique to their system. This leader can make change occur and is instrumental in not only continuing to have an organization that can innovate but mentoring newer leaders to lead in the system as well. There is so much change occurring, and change needs to occur at such a fast pace that this leader knows they cannot and should not be the one making all the decisions. The larger the system, the further this leader is from the product (the care provided to an individual), and the more external and

---

EXPERIENCE FROM THE FIELD

New Knowledge Driving Change at a System Level

As a Nurse Scientist, it is important to translate and utilize research findings in a meaningful way to make change. In a large health system, generating new knowledge or enacting a practice change can take advantage of the benefits that a system can offer. We conducted a multihospital evidence-based practice project to implement monthly gratitude practices in teams during the height of COVID-19 pandemic surges. The idea was sparked when the American Nurses Foundation and the Greater Good Science Center asked our health system to implement a gratitude toolkit they created. Rather than simply hand out the toolkit, we sought to measure outcomes. We formed a team of site champions and created a single EBP protocol and implementation plan. We also received a single Institutional Review Board (IRB) nonresearch determination. Each hospital utilized the protocol while still enjoying the autonomy of implementing unique to their culture. For example, one hospital chose to have a separate team formed to select gratitude practices and run the campaign, whereas another hospital chose to run the project through their shared governance. Each hospital gave their nurses a presurvey prior to implementing monthly gratitude practices that included measuring gratitude, flourishing behaviors, and mindfulness. For six months, site coordinators supported their hospital in conducting monthly gratitude practices, such as a gratitude wall, huddles, three good things, or a savoring walk. After six months, a postsurvey to nurses was conducted. With the help of the Nurse Scientist, results were analyzed and each facility was presented with a summary of findings and benchmarked results—making it meaningful to the site to see their own results in addition to the larger study. All the site leaders came together to present the study in a podium presentation and write a manuscript.

Lesly Kelly, PhD, RN

internal influences are influencing the outcome. Two of the most important job functions of a formal leader in a health care system are to decentralize decision-making and to hire the best leaders.

Some may argue that those two functions are important in any role in any type of organization. This is true, but based on what we know about systems, nursing, and patient outcomes, this becomes increasingly important in larger complex systems that tend to become more bureaucratic and hierarchal in nature as a result of growth and an attempt to organize the system. Remember that the RN roles we discussed earlier all have a piece of knowledge in the system that no one else has. No one can know everything; thus, it is vital that the experienced nurse manager and executive build and maintain a culture where the wealth of information can be shared and where everyone can be a part of the decision-making process.

Decision-Making in a System

The leader's role in creating and shaping such cultures is dependent on their ability to create the infrastructure and processes required to support a clinical enterprise based on a professional model of practice. In this model of the professional role, the RN is viewed and supported as a pivotal decision maker on the interdisciplinary team (Forsey & O'Rourke, 2013).

Decisions should be made by the staff closest to patient care. Quite often in shared leadership, managers either lead the discussion in the direction they want or

---

EXPERIENCE FROM THE FIELD

Another Nurse Leader's Style

For decades, I had worked in several health care systems and found significant advantages as a leader and as a professional. Early on in a large system, I was promoted to a mid-level leadership role in one of the smaller facilities, and this could have been an isolating and risky experience. However, quite quickly I learned I had a supportive and accessible group of colleagues who formally met on mutual projects while also being available informally to each other. Even though my new colleagues worked in multiple facilities in several states, through technology, we had ready access to each other. A deep and rich network is a distinct advantage of working in a system.

Colleen Hallberg, RN, MSN

later undo a decision made by the group. This happens most often because we are functioning within that bureaucratic structure. Staying out of the way and being clear from the onset of group or team work about what is in scope and out of scope not only empowers them but also demonstrates their leadership skills in addition to enhancing your own.

EXPERIENCE FROM THE FIELD

Being an informal leader throughout the COVID-19 pandemic, helping to support a team and watching other formal leaders, I have found a few things to be very applicable in the world of tele-health and in health care in general:

1. The changes to process and care delivery can be fast, and that is something we know happens in health care. We need to ensure communication channels are planned out before, and information needs to be delivered in a very direct and clear manner. Items should be reviewed by a member of the team BEFORE being sent out to the larger group, as a fresh set of eyes of someone who does the work can save a lot of time having to explain or reeducate something that was delivered incorrectly in the first place.

2. People need to feel heard and some-times just need to vent or it will impact their work. Take the time to allow people to do this, even if it means the metrics are a bit "off." People are more important than the metrics. INVEST in your team.

3. Frustrations with broken processes, the helpless feeling when you cannot do anything for a patient, patient

attitude, and lack of compassionate formal leaders are leading to signifi-cant moral injury for health care workers. This needs to be acknowl-edged and not just glossed over with canned responses.

4. A higher number of staff members were out on leave during the pan-demic, sometimes not COVID-19 related. Check in on your staff when they are out on leave and make it not related to return to work. A simple phone call or text can make a huge difference.

5. Get your hands dirty and know what your team members actually do. You cannot expect to be speaking to other leaders about the capacity of your team, especially in times of rapid change and crisis, if you do not have a good idea of the current realities and workflows.

6. As leaders, you are also experiencing moral injury and need to find ways to address it. You will be no good to everyone else if you are struggling yourself. This can cause team mem-bers to leave. It is very true that people more often leave a poor leader over frustrations with the actual job.

Jennifer Tucker, MA, RN

In being clear about scope, there may be instances during work when certain triggers may call for discussion with individuals with higher management authority. Not having clear boundaries for staff may lead to confusion, disappointment, and bad feelings toward the shared leadership structure. I like to call clear boundaries guardrails, which are a set of parameters within which the team can work freely. Within the guardrails, something can be developed and decisions can be made. If something goes beyond the guardrails or parameters, then the team will need to seek further assistance from a manager or go up the chain of command for approval before action can occur. A list of triggers to consider includes the following:

1. Issues with impact to the budget

2. Change in scope of practice

3. Change in scope of service for one facility that may affect others

4. Variance from strategic initiative expectation

5. Adding components to scorecard/initiative/measurements

6. Contract issues at a facility that may impact others

7. Decisions that have a significant impact on physician or employee relations

Guardrails or triggers should not be seen as areas one cannot cross but more as gray areas that need input from others outside of the shared leadership team. Ensuring shared leadership and decentralized decision-making should be the foundation in all organizations regardless of size. This should not undermine the role of the manager or executive in decision-making. As the manager, you have the knowledge and experience of rules, regulations, policies, and other practices that staff may not have. Your shared leadership team cannot determine pay practices for themselves. You, as the manager, know human resources rules and can explain to your staff why this is an inappropriate topic for shared leadership. Your job is to provide them your expertise in formal management knowledge while allowing them to exercise their expertise in professional practice decision-making that impacts clinical care.

Talent Mapping/Succession Planning in a Health Care System

With the impending retirement of baby boomers from the workforce, organizations are focusing on *succession planning* and growing their next level of leaders. Succession planning in health care is a relatively new concept. Although other industries have utilized the process, it is still not as mature in a hospital setting. As the process was introduced within the system, with over 20 acute care hospitals and physician practices in seven states, one of the challenges was ensuring the consistency of definitions and a standard process utilized in all areas of the organization.

Year 1 focused on process consistency and standardized definitions. The focus of the first year was simply introducing the concept, the purpose, value, and anticipated outcomes. As you can imagine, getting 3,000 people to define "high performers" and "high potential" in the same way was quite challenging. The consistency in terms and identification of the skills, behaviors, and experiences for all areas of the system came when the talent calibration sessions were conducted outside the four walls of each facility. As we brought all the acute care facility CEOs together to discuss their talent, we gained momentum in standardizing what it took to be a leader of the future within the organization.

Year 2 focused on follow-up action items between leaders and employees who were a part of the process as well as creating programs to address themes and trends identified during the talent mapping sessions.

Year 3 was when the magic started to happen. Employees saw people were being promoted because of someone discovering they aspired for greater responsibility. People were moving from their home facility to another facility for career advancement. This also had unintended consequences for the system. While the leadership development philosophy was investment in 100 percent of the employees in the system with a differential investment in high potentials and high performers, some employees started to interpret the outcomes of the talent mapping process as "if I don't state that I have aspirations of being in the C-suite, I will be left behind." That was not true; however, perception is reality. We needed to be certain that if someone wanted to be a bedside nurse, the organization celebrated that decision! Not everyone can or should feel they have to be in the C-suite—after all, there are only a few of those positions. So we started messaging the value of all employees at every level within the organization. Each leader needed to learn to provide more robust and comprehensive feedback as an outcome of the talent mapping process. This was a separate conversation from the annual performance review process.

The lessons learned are probably consistent with any other process—communicate, communicate, communicate. Involve those who will be impacted or touched by the process to garner support and buy-in and, most important, be open to ideas and modifications from your key stakeholders as the process matures.

Janice E. Ganann, MEd, ACC,
Managing Director, JLG and Associates, LL

Finding the Right Leaders in Your System

In addition to mentoring, precepting, and leading staff in your system, it is important to identify new leaders and leaders for different roles. In a health care system, the benefit of being large is the large pool of RNs who know the organization, know the culture, and can be mentored for additional leadership roles or formal management positions. However, many organizations and systems fail to take advantage of the pool of talented RNs around them. Creating a succession plan in your organization for nursing is extremely important. It ensures that you have a pipeline of leaders for your organization as change occurs as well as lets RNs know that the organization recognizes their work and talent within the organization. Nothing can be more disappointing to aspiring leaders than when an organization feels that they need to go outside the organization to find the right nurse leader.

In the succession planning for RNs, remember it is about leadership. It is not about the clinical knowledge of the RN in the area in which they will lead and manage. All too often, direct-care RNs feel as if the manager must have clinical skills and ability in the specialty of their department or unit. This is a clear misunderstanding of the role of a manager. We all have roles in our organization, as we all are leaders. However, the best thing for a nurse manager to be is not a clinician who can help with direct patient care but who can figure out resources so that the direct-care clinicians are never short-staffed. If the manager is not doing their role, then who is? In order to have a system work, everyone must function in their role. If you need a nurse manager for an intensive care unit, then maybe the nurse manager in the home care department might have the right skills to meet the challenges in that department. Think outside of the box in a system. You have a system of talent; do not self-impose any more boundaries than already exist!

Nursing Leaders for the Future

As of the publication of this book, there are approximately 4.4 million nurses in the US. COVID-19, recessions, and retirements all impacted shortages of direct-care clinicians and leaders. While we could talk about the impact this will have on the overall workforce and dive into an overall nursing shortage discussion, we will not go there. Where we need to go is leadership. We will have many of our older formal nurse leaders leave, creating what some have called a brain drain in leadership. The brain drain is not all about leadership itself but about the working knowledge of being a manager, about regulations, accreditation, employee relations, and other management activities. Too often we mix the terms "leader" and "manager" together, but in order to solve this issue, we need to clarify what our real concern is: is it a lack of leaders or a lack of managers?

I have heard two kinds of conversations on this. Being a younger experienced nurse leader, I am part of the older experienced nurse leaders' discussions and concerns. There are concerns on all sides, regardless of the generation, and we now have five generations in the workplace! As in most conversations, it is important to seek an understanding of differences and work together for a collaborative answer.

There are so many things we need to accomplish as nurse leaders and managers in the next 10 years as our experienced leaders and managers retire and more of our younger nurses become leaders and managers. The last thing we need to do is continue any us-versus-them beliefs. All nurses, regardless of the generation, are committed in the same ways to our profession and being leaders. We all have and will do it our own ways. We need to honor the legacy of those who came before us while allowing those after to forge a new path.

Sometimes we act as if there is a shortage of formal nursing management or executive positions, as if that was the only way to be a leader or to lead. There is so much work to be done, and we truly need everyone managing and leading from where they are to get us to where we need to be as a profession and to advance the health of our nation. *It is moments like this when we each must be a leader.* We know the story of nurses eating our young. This is more than nurses eating our young. So let us each change it. This change starts with each of you. If we want nurse leaders for the future, think about the moments you have had in which you could make or break one. Rise every nurse up.

Key Points

- You are a nurse. You are a leader. Step into it and own it.

- The transformational leadership style allows for the recognition of areas in which change is needed and guides change by inspiring followers and creating a sense of commitment.

- It is important to always look beyond our own discipline and industry to know what others are doing that can be of use to us.

- It is important that you ask for a preceptor and seek a mentor who can help you navigate the politics of a complex multilevel organization.

- All nurses, regardless of the generation, are committed in the same ways to our profession and to being leaders.

- If we want nurse leaders for the future, think about the moments you have had in which you could make or break one.

CHAPTER 7

Systems Thinking from an Individual Organization Up

A system is a network of interdependent components that work together to accomplish the aim of the system. A system must have an aim. Without an aim, there is no system.

—W. Edwards Deming

Systems thinking within your organization is not too different from thinking beyond your organization. Smaller systems are embedded or nested within larger systems. This is the opportunity to capitalize on the knowledge of others and standardize processes! You may be thinking that you cannot even get everyone on same page in the same department or organization, let alone beyond! The thing is, you will not get everyone on the same page. You can get most people to head in the right direction and follow standardized processes through communication and collaboration and in turn have excellent patient outcomes. Start with determining the desired outcomes. Despite our differences, most people want the same things, but how we get there is where we usually differ the most.

The difference between chapter 7 and chapter 8 is that this chapter will focus on the individual in a department or single organization working their way up and between levels, departments, or organizations, whereas chapter 8 is about how corporate or system employees work down levels, to the organizational and departmental levels. Remember, this is not about hierarchical power but (as noted in chapter 3) how things develop up and down through the many levels in any organization and system.

Communication within Organizations

It has been said that communication is the most important key to leadership success. Communication is important for all RNs at any level in an organization. As an organization grows, communication becomes a challenge. How does one get their voice heard from the point closest to patient care by those in more removed levels of the organization? And just as importantly, how does the person at the farthest points from direct patient care get their voice and messages heard?

Communication is a two-way street, though. It is not purely about being heard but about listening as well. Listening is a challenge in every organization, starting with individuals. What is the definition of communication? The Merriam-Webster online dictionary defines communication as "a process by which information is exchanged between individuals through a common system of symbols, signs, or behavior; personal rapport; information communicated: information transmitted or conveyed; a verbal or written message."

In our complex environment, if we only expressed ourselves, we would not be able to advance our health care system. Arguably, that is one of our biggest problems now. We need to learn how to exchange information, which is a two-way street! Stephen Covey (2004) notes that for the most part, "people do not listen with the intent to understand; they listen with the intent to reply" (p. 239).

Think back to the last conversation you had with someone. As soon as the other person started to talk, did you waste no time in your mind constructing your response, only to realize that you had not really heard (and thus not really understood) the remainder of what the other person said? Poor communication, from one side or both, can create mistrust and silos. To improve communication, teach and demonstrate good communication skills to everyone! Improved communication skills are not the latest or greatest email or social media platform. No matter how great the communication plan is, if we do not have the appropriate interpersonal communication skills, it will not work.

Communication in Your Department

Seemingly simple methods of communication can be the most effective. Remember, an innovation does not need to involve technology or be something never heard of before. It just needs to be the right idea at the right time.

Posting information where people can stop and have time to understand the communication is quite effective. However, if you are inconsistent with where you post information or the frequency of the postings, the effectiveness will be decreased. Standardization is great for everything, including communications.

Communication in Your Organization

When I was in nursing school, I remember having an "interpersonal communications" course in my entry RN program. Unfortunately, that program, like many others, decided to wrap the content into other classes to make room for other classes that were needed. Communication, both written and personal, is a vital part of nursing. Our people skills as nurses are the foundation to a therapeutic relationship with our coworkers and our patients. Interpersonal skills are the skills we use when we engage in face-to-face communication with one or more people. While written and verbal communication is important, it is just the tip of the overall way in which we communicate. We communicate more information using nonverbal signals, such as gestures, facial expressions, body language, and even our appearance.

If you need to communicate within your organization, you might be sending out a lot of emails and phone calls. But you are more likely to have in-person contact with others within your organization than you would with those from different organizations in your system. We will talk more about written communications in the next section, but let us focus a little more here on in-person communication.

In-Person Communication

In-person communication can happen one-on-one or in a meeting. When you are in person, your interpersonal communication is very important because you are communicating so much with body language, and it can be interpreted negatively! Such negativity can be interpreted as bullying. Bullying can come across in all forms of communication, and chances are, you are probably making at least one gesture that is associated with bullying behavior without even knowing it!

If you are in a group meeting for the first time and people do not know you, they will watch your body language to try to understand more about you. Group meetings can also be stressful and feel conformist and rigid. There are some things you can do to ease those feelings.

One Nurse's Approach to Communications

My nursing practice in a teaching hospital neonatal intensive care unit (NICU) included being the designated day charge nurse; therefore, I attended high-risk deliveries, assisted in births in the emergency department parking lot, directed patient care, was a certified Peripherally Inserted Central (PIC) line inserter and trainer for the electronic health record implementation, defined and updated evidence-based policies and procedures, and served on many hospital-wide committees.

After many years of direct care practice, I was recruited to be the Nurse Educator for the NICU. I knew from personal experience and the experiences of my colleagues that communication to the staff would be the major barrier. The policies and procedures, important announcements, survey results, Evidence Based Practice (EBP), National Patient Safety Goals, Joint Commission standards, accreditation visits, and educational offerings proved very difficult to communicate to every nurse, every shift, 24/7. There are various ways to communicate with all staff, personalizing to individual needs; however, there are issues with having various communication methods. Issues such as people not checking unit email, not participating in timely reporting, or not knowing where to look forced me to

develop a communication process in the one place I knew I could capture every nurse, every shift—the staff bathroom. I called the project the "Toilet Papers," but the name may not be considered appropriate for all settings. I posted every manner of critical information—information that was unit specific or hospital-wide, every topic that the NICU nurses (and physicians, medical and nursing students, and ancillary staff) needed to know. Certainly critical information was disseminated by email and other more mainstream methods, but in this way, topics could be introduced visually and prioritized for the NICU.

In the interest of not being serious all the time, I posted funny articles and tasteful cartoons depicting nurses and babies. No wall was left unutilized, and all documents were laminated prior to posting and cleaned daily. Postings remained for a minimum of one month in order to reach all staff, no matter how infrequent their practice schedule. Meeting the goal of increased staff awareness and communication, the Toilet Papers program received positive reviews and was replicated in other units. A visit from the chief nursing officer provided further validation for this method of communication.

Teresa Stone, BSN, RNC, PRP-CP

Texting

Text and chat apps have become a go-to for immediate response. There are positive and negative aspects to texting, and one should be aware of when to and when not to use this as a communication technique.

Positive considerations:

- Quick when need a response now

- Saves time over constructing an email

- Often text messages arrive faster than emails

- May be easier way to introduce a hard subject asking for follow-up meeting

Negatives considerations:

- Hard to convey emotion

- Decreases social connection

- Creates bad grammar and spelling habits (that spill over into email and other written communication)

- Delay causes misunderstandings (not being responded to immediately, leading to feeling ignored)

When texting or using chat features, there are a few things to consider before using it. First, think about your audience. What is the appropriate communication medium that should be used? Take into consideration various cultures and how they may communicate differently. Also, do not use all caps. It does imply anger or panic. Always reread before sending. Autocorrect has gotten the best of all of us,

---

THINGS TO CONSIDER

Principles for Social Media

With TikTok, Reels, Instagram, and others social media apps becoming a norm within our culture, it is important to recognize where one can get in trouble professionally with its use. A good go-to reference is the American Nurses Association's Social Media Principles found at https://www.nursingworld.org/social/.

replacing a misspelled word that could get anyone in trouble with human resources. And, as with emails, do not make them long.

Walking Meetings

One suggestion to improve communication in a small group meeting or even one-on-one meetings is to have walking meetings. This decreases issues with body language and improves the productivity of the meeting! Now, in a time when more individuals have work at home days or work remote completely, walking during meetings is gaining traction.

- The energy of walking makes you more alert . . . no one ever falls asleep in a walking meeting.
- Fresh air and light improve mental well-being.
- Walking side by side decreases "hierarchy" work distinctions.
- Getting you closer to the 10,000 steps a day goal for every person!

Sounds intriguing, but you do not know where to start. Here are some tips in conducting and being a part of successful walking meetings:

- Organize what you need, including an agenda, before the meeting.
- Make sure people know it is a walking meeting.
- Have the right shoes! Three-inch heels (or any inch heels!) are going to be distractingly painful.
- Consider weather: bring umbrellas if necessary.
- Schedule earlier in the day for warmer climates.
- Schedule in the afternoons if you need to meet at a time when people tend to get tired faster when sitting.
- Avoid busy roads and construction. Use sidewalks, parks, or walking trails.
- Walking meetings are best for small groups but, if planned well, could be used for a larger group.

- Wear an "I am on a Walking Meeting" badge so people who were not invited do not decide to join you.

- From home, buy a laptop table for your treadmill to walk at a 2-mph speed while meeting if face time is required.

You might be asking, with technology and our mobile society, why have a face-to-face meeting at all? After all, we need to save money in our health care system, and other methods work just as well. Well, not always. Consider a face-to-face meeting in the following situations:

- You need to have conversation off the record. Emails can be forwarded, and phone calls can be recorded. So can in-person meetings, but it is much less likely.

- You need to get to know each other first. Ice-breaking meetings are better in person. Then the work can be done after everyone has gotten a chance to know each other first.

- You want to get a sense of the environment and culture where others work.

- The meeting is over tough or sensitive material for which the ability to read body language would be beneficial.

- You are proposing a new idea and want to garner support.

- It is important for individuals to spend time learning about each other.

Best rule of thumb: If you are unsure about the type of meeting, make it a face-to-face one if possible. If not, set ground rules to require people to have cameras on while in virtual meetings. If individuals are remote, expectations in their job descriptions and positions should be that having cameras on should be the norm.

Body Language: Positive and Negative

You cannot escape the use of body language in society. I had a neighbor who was a used car salesperson. He taught me a body language tip that salesmen have been known to use. When you come in to discuss and negotiate the purchase of a car, you usually shake hands a few times in the process, such as at the beginning of negotiations. As the salesman goes to shake your hand, he might turn his wrist in, which places your palm up and his palm down. This is a very small, subtle sign to you that you are open to negotiations and he is not, even if he says otherwise. Here are some other tips for positive body language:

- Keep your movements relaxed.

- Use open arm gestures.

- Show the palms of your hands—this is a silent signal of credibility and candor (*I have nothing up my sleeves to hide*).

- Smile! People prefer happy people.

- Always have a firm handshake.

- Be aware of others' personal space and respect it.

- Have eye contact without staring.

- Nod when people talk (it helps them relax), but clarify if you do not understand or do not agree. I nod with people when I agree but also when I understand them.

To improve on my body language and verbal communication skills, I continue to work on them, one at a time. Not that I am now perfect; it is a journey. For instance, I would have a trusted coworker help me with the behavior I wanted to change, like saying "um" when I spoke. I have gotten good at never saying "um" when I talk, but we all know the person (yourself!) that is a big offender on this issue. Saying "um" distracts from the conversation and decreases your credibility. I would have the coworker help me count all the times I said "um," and my goal was to be at zero times in any meeting, which I believe I have met!

Then there are the unintended body language movements that people may interpret in ways that may surprise you! I had a coworker ask me if I was nervous and I asked why. He said that I was fidgeting with my paper coffee cup. I always get a mocha in the morning from a certain coffee shop, and by time I get down to the last 10 percent, the chocolate can settle at the bottom if they did not stir it right, so I would swirl the cup to mix it with the coffee. This coworker interpreted my swirling as being nervous! I appreciated it greatly that he asked me instead of assuming.

Having a coworker or friend help you with your body language will make a positive impact on your communication style. These are individuals you see on a regular basis, and they can help you be the best you! Here are some other tips on avoiding negative body language: When we are nervous or stressed, we tend to engage in nervous fidgeting, such as rubbing our hands together, bouncing our feet, drumming our fingers on the desk, or playing with our jewelry. All of these are distractions from the intended communication. If I found that if I had started to do any one of these, I would subtly move my hands to my seat and sit on them until I relaxed. I also may lightly sit on my hands as a reminder to myself to not talk so much and to allow others to talk. Listening more than we talk is an important aspect of being a leader.

Additionally, consider these body movements when trying to keep communication open and positive:

- Do not point with your finger. If you must point, use your knuckle.

- Do not cross your arms.

- Do not roll your eyes.

- Do not sigh.

All of these body movements are considered a type of bullying.

Communication between Organizations

Written Communication

Written communication happens a lot. Probably too much! While there are downfalls to in-person communication, like bad body language, no body language is probably even worse for creating issues in communication! Setting the smiling faces and other emoticons aside, it is still hard to interpret written messages like emails, especially if you do not know the writer. Some people have different senses of humor, which can be taken badly, or they might cut right to the chase in an email, which can seem cold and callous.

When you are in a system, you probably are not driving to each meeting. Nor should you have to, as it takes a lot of time and money to drive. Some things can be taken care of via email or conference call.

However, be mindful of long email chains! Once an email chain has three responses and the issue or question is not resolved, stop emailing. The fourth email should be one that states the "conversation is going offline" and that the appropriate conference call or in-person meeting will be scheduled to further discuss and resolve the issue at hand. Nothing creates more confusion than long email chains, which may or may not have all the emails in it depending on if a recipient replied to all or just the original sender. It takes a lot of skill to successfully manage any email conversation, let alone resolve a major issue via email.

While the tips to improve communication skills can be used for verbal and in-person communication, they are also very helpful for written communication. When communicating via email, consider the following tips to improve your sender and recipient skills. Many times in a health care system, you might not know the person with whom you are communicating. Or perhaps you have only ever had a virtual working relationship. When I worked in a multiple state system, I had emailed with someone for years to accomplish different tasks yet had never seen them! In two health care systems, employee pictures were posted online for people to see on a large system organizational chart, as well as in the email system. This helped people "get to know" virtual coworkers better.

So, what types of communication should be via email? Although it cannot and should not replace all face-to-face communication and other forms of communication, emails can be an effective method for sharing basic information, such as new cafeteria prices, security precautions, or prework and the agenda for an in-person meeting. Emails, if set up appropriately, can also let people know who looked and did not look at an email.

THINGS TO CONSIDER

A Tip on Emoticons

There can be as many as five generations working in the same place, and each of us has a different perspective on appropriate and inappropriate communication styles. Rule of thumb, if you do not know someone well, you probably should not be using emoticons in your email or messaging apps. They can be interpreted as unprofessional or, worse, misinterpreted as meaning something other than what was intended to someone who is not skilled in emoticon interpretation.

While they are gaining popularity, generational differences of emoticons can cause issues. What I as a Gen X individual may think an emoticon may mean may in fact have a different meaning to a different generation! I think about words I used as a teen/ young adult. Those words are used very differently by my Gen Z children!

Here is a list of dos and don'ts for using email:

- The email should be concise and to the point, not three or more paragraphs on a regular basis.

- Use plain text and common fonts with a simple signature line. Fancy graphics, fonts, and backgrounds can take up unnecessary storage space in the recipient's inbox and may load slowly or not at all, especially on people's smartphones.

- Stick to one topic in the email and write only the things that are appropriate for anyone to read, as email forwarding makes it possible for originally unintended parties to receive the email.

- Proper grammar and spelling are very important because they reflect on you and your abilities. Turn on grammar and spell check for your emails and use it. It will not fix everything, but it is a start.

- Never use text slang or shorthand in an email or any work communication.

- Attachments should be prepared in a format that any recipient can easily access/download. If only limited people have Visio in the organization, then sending something saved in Visio will keep some people from looking at it. Save any file like a Visio to a PDF and then send.

- Do not use BCC unless you tell the person you are BCC'ing first. Better yet, just forward the message to them in a separate email. I have seen people

---

A CONSIDERATION FOR SYSTEMS THINKING

Tips to Improve Communication

General skills:

- Clarify the goal of the communication.

- Anticipate the recipients' feelings and how your message may be received.

- If there is an action to be undertaken, clearly call that out.

- Clearly note any deadlines or time-frames in the subject line of an email or on an agenda.

- Confirm the recipients' understanding.

Listening skills:

- Keep an open mind.

- Clarify any part that is unclear.

- Confirm your understanding.

mysteriously show up in a conversation because they received the email but did not realize they had only been BCC'd.

- If an email makes you upset, put it aside. Come back and respond once you have reconciled your emotions, or once you have calmed down, pick up the phone. It is just a miscommunication!

- Use an SBAR format (Situation, Background, Assessment, Recommendation) to write up an email when you are asking or needing something.

A mentor once told me that information is just information. It is not "good" or "bad"; it is just information. What makes it good or bad is how we react to it. If you want to label something bad or not good, make sure you understand the full message correctly. Think through why you are reacting the way you are as well. Then back to the last tip: Do not send an emotion-packed email! Work to understand, not anger, others. Organizations have their own long memories, as do the people who work in health care systems. Employees have a tendency to move around in different positions. You want to be known as the great communicator, not the emotional one!

Virtual Meetings

Even though everyone should have cameras on for virtual meetings, technology and the Internet may not always be cooperative. Virtual meetings do not need to always have video to be successful. Otherwise known as a conference call or teleconferencing, they just take a good understanding of communication skills to navigate! This type of meeting can be interesting to attend and to chair. An unintended positive for this type of meeting is that the shy attendees are more likely to participate in this type of meeting. However, it is also harder to stop people from talking too much!

Tips for successful conference calls are the following:

- Prepare before with setting a formal agenda and send out all the material ahead of time so people can prep for call (do not send the hour before; send it a few days ahead!).

- Label handouts appropriately and use the labels to help people figure out what is being looked at.

- Take a roll call, and keep track of who is on the call.

- Encourage participation: If you haven't heard from someone, ask if they have something to say.

- Be on time. Nothing is worse than people joining 5 to 10 minutes late.

- Place your phone on mute, especially if you are at home, in the car, or in your office. Background noise like dogs barking and coworkers stopping by is disruptive.

- Place a sign on your office door that says you are in a phone meeting.

- Do not let any one person monopolize the call.

- Silence on the line feels even longer than in person, but allow it so that people can think, reflect, and prepare a response.

- Stick to the agenda—add a timeframe to each piece to keep on track.

- Keep minutes and record the call.

- Make sure people know each other on the phone and complete an introduction if people do not know each other.

- Ask the people to disclose if others are on the phone with them.

- If you are late to the call, announce yourself as soon as possible. Few things are worse than finding out a member of the team was listening the entire time and no one knew it. Sending an email or instant message to the leader to announce your arrival may work well.

Virtual meetings can be an efficient and effective way to meet. It takes an organized chair to run a meeting successfully, but attendees are an important part of making the meeting work well!

Collaboration within Organizations

In your health care system, to standardize, innovate, and improve patient outcomes, you need to collaborate. Collaboration goes hand in hand with effective communication. But why collaborate at all? Because no one, no matter how smart they are, knows everything, even the expert!

Remember bounded rationality from the introduction? With representation on teams, whether to improve operational functions or patient care, collaboration brings various viewpoints together so that we can decide with the best understanding of the issue as a whole.

Collaboration is working jointly with others. However, just working together does not mean you are collaborating. You could just be cooperating or coordinating (Winer & Ray, 1994). Real collaboration requires a commitment to shared goals, a jointly developed structure and shared responsibility, mutual authority and accountability for success, and the sharing of resources, risks, and rewards. As the name suggests, this is not a top-down, hierarchical structure or process but a joint endeavor. If this was a hierarchical process, then we would call it cooperating or coordinating.

So, what does collaboration look like from your health care system level? There are four keys to successful collaboration (Murray, 2017). As a team is formed, these are important items to get group clarity on:

1. *Clarify the purpose:* What are you trying to accomplish?

2. *Let form follow function:* Choose the simplest form possible to accomplish your goal.

3. *Involve the right people:* Involve the fewest people possible, but cover all viewpoints.

4. *Get it in writing:* Create, maintain, and update a charter. An absolute must!

All of this should be stated in the charter created. If you have never used a charter, ask if your organization has a template for one. If not, there is a sample in this book (see appendix). Write up the charter, share with the team, and ask for input. Bring it to every meeting, and update it as needed. Your team may have multiple levels of employee involvement. So let us talk about how we can improve collaboration based on those four items at different levels of your organization.

Collaboration in Your Department

Collaboration might seem easiest if done within your own department or unit. There may be differences in opinions, priorities, and goals within your area; however, they are usually focused on the same end point. Everyone in your department may have their own ways of getting to that goal. The best way to accomplish a goal in a department is through shared leadership.

Many units, departments, and organizations have some form of shared leadership (or shared governance, as it is called as well). Shared leadership is leadership that is broadly distributed, so that people within a unit, a department, and/or an organization lead each other.

The key to this level of shared leadership and collaboration is that you do not and cannot invite the entire staff to be involved. As noted earlier, keep the team smaller. The larger the team, the more likely you will not be able to come to a consensus on items, which will slow you down.

When it comes to purpose, make sure that everyone is clear on this and that it is communicated clearly to nonmembers of the team.

Well-intentioned members may want to solve all of the problems in the department, which is something we call scope creep. You jeopardize the original intent and goal by not focusing on a detailed plan and timeline to solve the issue at hand. Remember, you can always create a team to solve the other issue(s). Just do not try to do it all at once. Creating a charter helps avoid scope creep as all members can see the goal, timeline, and deliverables. If someone suggests something that involves scope creep, then you can point out the charter and use the charter to guide inclusion or exclusion of the item.

Collaboration in Your Organization

Collaboration in the larger setting of the organization can take on a shared leadership role as well. However the team is set up, having the right people at this level really starts to provide a positive impact on your outcomes.

Again, this is not about including everyone and making people feel included. This is about getting a goal accomplished through collaborating with the right players. There will be people who feel that they should be on a team, not because of what they can bring to the discussion but because they have controlling personalities.

How do you pick the right people without picking everyone? Here are some things to consider in choosing members for the team. These could apply at the unit/department level; however, they become more relevant at an organizational level.

- *Best fit for the role:* Think about knowledge and capability. A tough call might be between the seasoned employee who is truly knowledgeable but jaded and the newer employee who is less knowledgeable but full of passion and excitement.

- *Best fit for the team:* You do not want people who will not participate or who will just go along with whatever the group decides. You need active participation and individuals who are known to be collaborative. You do not want to bring on someone who will stall and deteriorate the collaborative abilities of others.

- *Good communicators:* If there are issues arising, you want people to bring them up and place them at the table for discussion. Having an elephant in the room stalls communication and in turn stops a collaborative environment.

- *The best connectors:* Depending on the issue, this can be more or less important. Who has the most connections in the organization that they can bring a systems perspetive to the team? This is usually the person who knows people beyond their own department.

- *Representative:* Does this committee reflect diversity, inclusion, and equity (DEI)? Having a team or group that represents DEI encourages diverse thinking, helps to reduce unconscious bias, and promotes accountability among many positives. Look around at the members. Are they people who look and think like you? If so, go back and select different members.

Once you have picked the members, clarifying roles is an absolute must. Unclear or overlapping roles can create conflict. Clearly define responsibilities, tasks, and goals that will populate the charter so that every member sees this and is clear about their role.

Collaboration in a health care department, unit, or organization is also about direct patient care between providers. If we are to provide care across the continuum, collaboration is necessary between not just nurses but all health care providers. Many things (silos, culture, ignorance, etc.) create barriers to successful collaboration to devastating effect. There is increasing evidence that coordinating care by assigning teams of providers can help reduce medical errors and improve quality, as well as help providers provide patient-centered, higher-quality care to an increasingly diverse patient population (RWJF, 2011).

To improve collaboration, it has been suggested that all health care professionals be taught to

- Assert the values and ethics of interprofessional practice

- Leverage the unique roles and responsibilities of interprofessional partners

- Communicate with patients, families, communities, and other health professionals

- Perform effectively in various team roles (Interprofessional Education Collaborative Expert Panel, 2011)

Collaborating with Similar Departments across the System

The complexity of collaborating comes in full force once you go beyond your own organization. Collaboration across similar departments might have a goal to standardize care guidelines for a certain patient diagnosis or to create standardized policies and procedures. As a system becomes more of a system, you want to reduce redundancies, improve appropriate standardization, and create a streamlined approach to care so that the patient does not see or receive different levels of care at different organizations in the system.

Here, understanding the end point or goal is key. Once you know the direction of the goal, team membership can start. As mentioned earlier, the right people

---

EXPERIENCE FROM THE FIELD

Individual Empowerment: Bottom-Up Drive for DEI

In my role as Director of Care Management, I was able to co-build an inclusive environment with my Black, Indigenous, and People of Color (BIPOC) staff. Early in 2020, several of my BIPOC staff asked if they could create a BIPOC support group that would also help bring to light structural and institutional racism within the department. I welcomed the idea, and this group started to meet on a regular monthly basis during paid time.

It was important for me to pay them for their time, and I managed my budget to cover costs of the team. During this time, we created a process to ensure one to two BIPOC clinicians were at all group interviews for new staff. We updated job descriptions that required hospital experience to instead allow for a diversity of experiences in settings with marginalized populations instead of hospital experience. I learned during this time that marginalized professional populations have a hard time becoming employed in a hospital setting, as they do not get the initial experience they need to meet requirements for better-paying hospital positions. This led to improved relationships with BIPOC clinicians who did not feel safe within our organization and to feel more welcomed.

Jennifer Mensik Kennedy,
PhD, MBA, RN, NEA-BC, FAAN

Collaboration from across the System

I had been working as a telehealth nurse, providing remote monitoring for patients with heart failure. Our home health agency and telehealth program had a strong relationship with our system's heart hospital, providing a continuum of care for patients with heart failure discharging from the acute setting. The heart hospital applied to be a Heart Failure Accredited Organization, which at that time would have made it the seventh hospital in the country to achieve this prestigious distinction. The process of becoming accredited required gathering several team members to submit documents that support the different domains: hospital, clinician, community, and science. Our agency and telehealth were part of the community domain. There were multiple others that were part of this committee to pull this all together, including physicians, the CEO, chief nursing officer (CNO), nursing directors of various departments, an insurance representative, social workers, and a mentor from the Accreditation Colloquium organization.

Our homework was to put together a packet of information from our assigned domain over the course of several months that showed process and supporting policies to satisfy accreditation requirements. We met multiple times over several months and discussed how our projects were coming along to meet the common goal of accreditation.

I learned several things over the course of those months. The most important thing I learned was that in a project as important as this, it is vital to follow instructions and not deviate! The directions of how to put our packets together were very meticulous. This was an example of a situation where if one person failed, the entire accreditation would have not been awarded. This distinction was important not only to the hospital but also to the larger hospital system and the community at large. I was not going to be the weak link. One initial direction our mentor gave us when we were putting together our individual packets was to put as much as possible into flowcharts. Having been in the clinical realm and not in any type of administrative role, I was not proficient with Visio and had to lean on our administrative assistant to assist me with putting our home health and telehealth processes into Visio flowcharts. In the end, when our packets were reviewed, our home health and telehealth packets were given a gold star for our flowcharts!

A second lesson I learned was that when you have multiple players who have a lot of decision-making abilities and very busy schedules (CEO, CNO, VP insurance company, physician) all at one table, there are many different agendas going on. There has to be one leader to redirect when you have deadlines. In our case, we did have important deadlines, or the accreditation was going to fall through. Our meetings at times tended to go off on tangents as everyone wanted to use that time when everyone was together to discuss other issues. Thankfully, our CEO had good relationships with everyone and took things offline when needed so that we were able to meet deadlines.

Susan Salo, BSN, RN

are very important to a collaborating team. When leading a team such as this, it is important to set expectations with members. Ensure that members can share their local best practices, but contribute in creating a new process with equal input from all. In groups, people often think that they need to talk everyone into doing it their way. Their organization is the best, right? Their patients are different, or sicker. Someone will always find a reason to not want to compromise and collaborate.

The goal in this level of collaboration should be on patient care outcomes and less on protecting one's own organization. For instance, a team of medical nurses is coming together to standardize heart failure care standards. Each team member should come in as organization A's expert in medical heart failure care first, not just as a nurse representing the individual facility's interest.

How Your Department Fits into the Bigger Picture

As we move further into collaboration across the system, what does this look like and how do we collaborate effectively? Take, for instance, the heart failure RNs mentioned in the previous section. What if it was more than standardizing care at hospitals but rather standardizing care across the continuum? Who is the expert there? Each representative is an expert in their area and brings the unique perspective of their setting to the table. Remember that no one person knows everything. Working together collaboratively helps to guide us in providing the best care for the patient, instead of protecting our own individual interests.

Your Role on an Organization or Systemwide Team

Getting a diverse representative team in any organization or system is no easy feat. The hardest part for many individuals or organizations is *trust*. Trust in each other so that you do not need multiple people from the same department or service line or organization to ensure appropriate representation. What you need is to clarify the role of any individual on a team. In the next chapter, I will discuss how you can go about picking the individuals once you determine the appropriate group size! What types of teams can be systemwide?

- Service line-based teams representing cardiology services from each facility

- Nursing shared leadership representing nursing from each organization

- Care coordination teams that represent different stages across the continuum to inform patient handoffs

A team is a group of people who come together for a common purpose. A group in and of itself does not necessarily constitute a team. Teams should have members with complementary skills that, through a coordinated effort, will allow each member to contribute positively toward the goal of the team. A team is not a group of people who all have their own vested interest in the goal and want to make sure the outcomes go their own way.

While shared leadership and teams work at being inclusive and sharing decision-making, it is possible to lose the benefit of the team if the team is too large. This then turns a team into a group of people who have their own reasons for attending or who may not even attend at all! We all know these "teams," the ones with one person who does all the talking, one who says it cannot be done, one who never does the work before showing up to the team meeting, one who does not show up at all, and one who shows up but looks at their email the entire time!

The appropriate size with the right team members is dependent on the type and purpose of the team. Current science around effective team size suggests around 5 and no more than 10 people; however, when the team is a representation of something larger, such as different organizations, teams may be upward of 18 to 20 individuals. The teamwork principles of accountability and cohesiveness that are necessary to achieve high performance become difficult as teams grow. Therefore, work to keep teams under 12 for sure. Ensure that individuals understand their role as part of the team. Individual member responsibilities may include the following:

- Bring your knowledge and ability regarding the team's work to the table.

- Do not protect or think only of your unit, department, or organization.

- Contribute to systems thinking.

- Work collaboratively with chair or team lead and other team members.

- Support ideas and changes within the unit or facility that the team agrees upon.

- Identify barriers and/or concerns that will hinder progress.

- Stick to and help in managing timeline, deliverables, and goals.

- Attend every meeting, show up on time, and stay for the entire meeting (if unable to attend, discuss with the chair or team lead if a substitute is needed in your place for that meeting).

- Check and respond to email and other communication or information methods in a timely manner.

Leading in a system from the organizational level up involves great communication and collaboration. Nurses at each level in any type of organization need to be involved in change and innovation, but that does not mean every nurse needs to be involved in every decision each time or things might not get done. Having the right nurse at the right time can make a difference between a team meeting their goals or not. All teams should have an end point. Having deliverables, goals, and timelines will ensure everyone understands their role and expectations on the team.

Key Points

- Communication is a two-way street.

- Collaboration is not a top-down, hierarchical structure or process but a joint endeavor.

- Diversity, equity, and inclusion are necessary for an inclusive bottom-up approach.

- It is necessary to have clearly defined responsibilities, tasks, and goals in the charter so that every member sees them and is clear about their role.

- The teamwork principles of accountability and cohesiveness that are necessary to achieve high performance become difficult as teams grow.

CHAPTER 8

Systems Thinking from the Corporate Office Down

Authority without wisdom is like a heavy axe
without an edge; fitter to bruise than polish.

—Anne Bradstreet, American poet

Organizational growth, particularly through mergers or acquisition, can be an
unsettling time for many employees. Naturally, all employees may wonder: Can the
organization sustain this growth? Will I lose my job? Will my job change? Who will
I report to? What kind of leader are they? Will they start telling us to do our jobs
differently? As the health care environment evolves and more health care organizations become a part of a system, whether or not as accountable care organizations
(ACOs), these questions become important to recognize and resolve before anxiety
can do any damage.

As we have learned in prior chapters, it is normal for organizations to become
more bureaucratic and hierarchical as they grow, to manage the complexity. But
how do we keep the need to create a structure in all the chaos from dictating and
driving decision-making from the top down?

When I was a system-level corporate employee, undoubtedly others saw me as a
decision maker, the one who told everyone else what to do as related to clinical
practices. However, I knew my role to be different and worked to demonstrate that
difference. My goal as a member of the system (in this case, a corporate employee)

was not to make all the decisions that would trickle down but to be the support person for all the facilities related to clinical practices, to be the person who bridged the gaps between the units, departments, facilities, and the system. My goal was to support the individual facilities, not to have the individual facilities support me.

When I say "support" here, I mean that my position was to make individual organizations' lives easier, to get things done that they needed help with. My role was to remove barriers and to facilitate systems thinking to set up committees for success. Again, those who knew what needed to be done to provide the best patient care are those closest to it. The support I did expect from an individual facility was the support of systemwide decisions, which in most cases were made by individuals representing each individual organization across the system.

In this chapter, we will discuss the role of the corporate or system employee in the health care system. Whether you are a direct-care nurse in a home care agency or the nurse executive, it is important to understand this role.

We will also discuss the issues with top-down and bottom-up approaches in decision-making and how to navigate these potential issues in addition to how to work on system-level team development.

Goals at Different Levels

Facility Specific and Systemwide

Everyone wants to do the right thing. Everyone also sees how to do the right thing their own way. In an individual facility, there could be multiple organizational personalities or subcultures. Some individual organizations will do what they need to do to play fairly with other organizations and are very collaborative, while others feel they are too different (often an excuse with no data to back it up) or feel that their way to success is not in toeing the corporate line but in being the rebels. You can imagine the trickledown effect that has within each organization, especially when requesting individuals to be on system-level teams. Employees play out and are representatives of their organization's culture.

The goal of an individual facility is to meet or exceed the goals set for them through strategic planning. Systemwide goals and planning vary depending on the maturity of the system as a whole. Some systems may partner with an individual organization to create facility-specific goals, while others may create a systemwide mandate that all organizations must meet regardless of the organizations' starting points! Needless to say, how the goals are developed has an effect on the outcomes achieved. Most people want to achieve their goals, and an organization is no different.

Goals of the Corporate Office

The goal of the corporate office, based on systemwide strategic planning, is to ensure that system goals, and therefore individual goals, are met. How can everyone succeed, and how do we monitor everyone and help everyone succeed, even if an organization does not want help? Managing relationships and ensuring outcomes across organizations without direct authority is a tough job, and not everyone is cut out to do it. This type of leader knows how to motivate and make change without having any authority! This takes a skilled leader. Where a manager might use heavy-handed authority to reinforce change, a corporate leader should be very thoughtful in their leadership approach for accomplishing outcomes.

Systemwide Efficiencies and Effectiveness: Communication and Collaboration

One main goal or desired outcome of a system is to become more efficient and effective within each individual organization but also as a system that delivers care along the continuum. Organizations may become part of another system because they are driven by a belief that there is a value in the relationship that has a positive outcome. Becoming more efficient and effective is a common outcome as organizations come together and start to act like a system. Standardization of processes is one way to achieve this and improve patient outcomes. Effective standardization requires collaboration. There are some negatives about being a system that everyone should aware of, such as partial loss of individual organization or unit identity, but this should not stop organizations from forming systems.

The key is to understand the concerns of the individuals in the facility but also the patients and people an organization serves in the community. Communication and partnerships should build on making alliances at all levels and alleviating concerns. Things to consider from the view point of patients and individual facility employees:

- Concern that health care prices will rise
- Concern that they will lose their voice

- Concern that priority on profits will come before care

- Concern that staffing levels will decrease

Ensuring great communication and collaboration can offset some of these concerns and over time build trust and a brand in the community. Unintentionally, in a health care system, top-down models and structures can inadvertently create issues for communication and collaboration. It is important to understand at the system level the impact you have and when to think about the system and the facility, as well as the individual patient! Despite being part of a system, there is always a culture and a context at each organization that needs to be understood and taken into consideration.

Bottom-Up Approaches: Recognizing the Atomistic Fallacy

While it is true that there are many issues with a top-down approach with mandates to individual facilities, this does not mean that a bottom-up approach is always ideal. Going back to the individual organization, there are times when a bottom-up approach (very decentralized approach) to making change can be negative. I have mentioned throughout this book that we need decentralized models, and the people closest to the patient need to be involved in decision-making. However, the method used at a department or unit level that works well may not work well if replicated elsewhere or facility-wide! In multilevel thinking, there are potential organizational issues known as atomistic and ecological fallacies. Whether you are in an individual organization or are a system corporate employee, having a basic understanding of both will allow you to make the best decisions on how to lead in the system.

The Atomistic Fallacy and Organizational Perspective

An *atomistic fallacy* can occur when one makes inferences about groups or aggregates from individuals or individual-level data. Issues can arise when making this type of inference because associations between two variables at the individual level may differ from associations between similar variables measured at the group level (Diez Roux, 2002). An inference is a conclusion reached based on evidence and reasoning. However, the conclusion reached is based on making the wrong assumptions from the evidence. You could also say these types of conclusions could be made based on faulty reasoning. Whew! That was a complex definition, but a system is complex, even at the level of two variables.

A well-known example of an atomistic fallacy concerns a study of individuals that finds that increasing individual-level income is associated with decreasing coronary heart disease mortality. It could be inferred then (or extrapolated) from these data that at the country level (like the US), increasing per capita income is associated with decreasing coronary heart disease mortality. However, this inference is wrong when looking at country-level data. Here the individual making this inference would be committing an atomistic fallacy. Actual data show that across many countries, increasing per capita income may actually be associated with increasing coronary heart disease mortality (Diez Roux, 2002). So you can see, there must be other variables at play at the individual level besides income, variables that play a role in decreasing coronary heart disease mortality that are not captured when inferred at a higher level. At what point did the inference become an atomistic fallacy? You would have to look at the data for the individual, town or county, state, and national levels to determine that.

From an individual- or organizational-level perspective, it may seem that if a process is working well and obtaining the right outcomes, we would want to share and replicate this process across other departments, facilities, and the system. However, this assumption is an atomistic fallacy. Specifically, this is where the compilation type of emergence described in chapter 3 comes in handy. A concept at an individual level may be different from its counterpart at a higher level, however similar the situation may seem. Just taking a best practice from one area and applying it to an entire facility does not guarantee success. Worse yet, since leaders may not understand the principles of an atomistic fallacy, managers who are not successful at rolling out a process that worked well elsewhere but fail to get similar results may be penalized as poor leaders and managers when that may not be the case. No matter how great a leader, some things will not work outside of the context in which they were developed.

Later on, I will discuss the other fallacy, ecological. But for now, note both types of fallacies are due in part to the complexities of the environment in which our system operates. As noted earlier, health care systems are open systems, and there are always changes going on. Different viewpoints and knowledge are needed at each level to ensure goals are met in this ever-evolving world! Think of the idiom, "they couldn't see the forest for the trees." In a health care system, no one knows everything, and those at the individual facility level are more likely to just see the trees. This is fine; it is their point of view and they are experts in trees. On the flip side, the corporate office is supposed to see the bigger picture; they are involved in

We Are Different: Allowing for Differences When They Do Exist

Over the years, I have worked in five health care systems covering one to multiple states. Early on, we learned that all players had to be represented in the decision-making process.

Emailing documents crafted by physicians in one state to a physician in another state, asking them to review and give input with a caveat that "no response means acceptance," did not guarantee buy-in by any stretch of the imagination. The best solution was either a visit or phone call from a physician leader when it was convenient for the practicing provider to actually discuss the proposal.

Then things got done.

My most valuable lesson has been to acknowledge that sometimes the excuse "We're different" is reality. Not "Our patients are different or sicker," which is rarely the case, but that the size of an institution, or its location, does impact its ability to comply with certain edicts from on high. By and large, leaders in facilities really do want to do what is best and safest for the patient and staff. They welcome change that adds value. That said, creating a system policy or care guideline that requires a pharmacist to review a prescription at 3:00 a.m. or an emergency department tech to accompany a laboring woman to Labor and Delivery (L&D) is an impossibility at a 35-bed rural hospital that may have only two RNs in house at 3:00 a.m. and no pharmacist or emergency department tech in sight. Successful systems learn to develop principles and standards that provide a homogeneous foundation of practice but leave the "how" of making it a reality up to the individual organization based on their state regulations and facility limitations.

System leaders need to listen to those in the trenches where the rubber meets the road and move away from the "father knows best" approach. While it is true that larger facilities generally bring more cash to the system, the size of the organization should not dictate whether we pay attention to their concerns or input. If we do not value and intend to listen to them, then do not invite them to join the system. As leaders, our intent should be to improve patient safety and provide the best care for every patient.

We do that by assisting them in developing practices that improve patient outcomes, not by loading providers and staff with bureaucratic red tape that does not add value to the challenges they already face.

Janne Sexton Taubman,
RN, MHA, MSN, FACHE

all the facilities, and their expertise lies in overseeing the larger forest. The problem corporate employees may have is that they cannot see the trees for the forest.

Corporate Collaboration with Facility Employees

As a corporate employee, it is important to know that while you might have been hired for your expertise in a subject, you are not the only expert. And furthermore, no one person can know everything. Collaboration and respect for individuals at the facility level are a must to be successful. Be a leader in the system helping people get their carrots, not a manager in the system holding the stick.

Top-Down Approaches: Recognizing the Ecological Fallacy

In a health care system, the corporate office is usually tasked with collecting all the information from every site in every possible way to be used in process and quality improvement activities, as well as research. This does have its benefits! Data collection is usually standardized, and measures are typically defined similarly. Then, with this large amount of data, outcomes can be compared appropriately, and information can be gleaned for furthering standardized processes that can be rolled out to organizations and departments. While this can be done and it sounds great, remember appropriate standardization? We need to ensure that the standardizations are appropriate before we roll anything out if we are expecting success. It is a common misconception that the larger the sample size, the better you will be statistically. This is true, to the point that you obtain the appropriate level of power statistically. There is such a thing as too much of a good thing with sample size! And now health care is among other industries that have what has been termed "big data." There are many things that need to be understood and taken into consideration prior to using big data to drive change. I will explain big data first before going into ecological fallacy.

Big Data: A New Solution and Issue in Systems Thinking

"Big data" is the latest buzzword in every industry, not just health care. Biology, physics, meteorology, and other areas have looked toward big data to solve outstanding questions in the world. *Big data* can be defined as data sets whose size or type is beyond the ability of traditional relational databases to capture, manage, and process. Furthermore, characteristics of big data include high volume, high velocity and high variety (IBM, 2023). In 2012, the Obama administration announced the Big Data Research and Development Initiative, which explored how big data could be used to address important problems faced by the government (Kalil, 2012). The initiative is composed of 84 different big data programs spread across six departments (White House, 2014).

Then, in 2016, the White House released the Federal Big Data Research and Development Strategic Plan. The plan included seven strategies that focused on advancing human understanding in all branches of science, medicine, and security; ensuring the nation's continued leadership in research and development; and enhancing the nation's ability to address pressing societal and environmental issues facing the nation and the world through research and development (Big Data, 2016).

You may have heard of a few of these programs, which include the National Security Administration (NSA) and its issues around lack, or even invasion, of privacy.

In addition to security issues and privacy concerns, big data may also introduce new problems, such as the *multiple comparisons* problem. When different individuals simultaneously test a large set of hypotheses, it is likely to produce many false results that mistakenly appear to be significant. The use of big data in science neglects statistical principles such as choosing a representative sample (as opposed to sample number based on a power analysis) because operators are too concerned about actually handling the huge amounts of data (Boyd, 2010). This approach may lead to results biased in one way or another, and it is a false premise to think that the larger the data set, the more likely your results are to be correct. Actually, what can happen is the opposite, where a type I error occurs. For those

How Much Data?

There are so much data and knowledge generated that the world's technological per capita capacity to store information has roughly doubled every 40 months since the 1980s (Hilbert & Lopez, 2011). And, as of 2012, every day 2.5 exabytes ($2.5 \times 1{,}018$) of data are created (International Business Machines [IBM], 2014).

who prefer not to remember their statistics course(s), a type I error represents a false positive, which leads one to conclude that a supposed effect or relationship exists when in fact it does not.

Considerations for Using Big Data

Big data can be very beneficial in a health care system and for patient care. It is important to understand that like anything, if big data are not well understood, issues can arise from the lack of understanding. I have been in meetings where big data were presented and decisions were made concerning major patient care changes, with a fundamental lack of understanding about the weaknesses in the data analysis. You do not need a PhD to understand the issues. As a leader, you need to be aware of these issues to raise crucial questions and be a critical thinker, not always a group thinker.

In chapter 4, I mentioned a quote by Dr. Farzad Mostashari, who said that "data is the oxygen for innovation." Why are data so important for innovation? "It is the key commodity that we need to be able to create new products, to be able to understand health better, [and] to bring the tools of data to health care" (Mostashari, 2014). So, ensuring your data are not only correct but also being applied correctly is vital in achieving successful innovation and outcomes.

Managing big data is an issue not only for organizations and systems but large databases as well. The federal government is looking at ways in which artificial intelligence (AI) can help manage and use large data sets. For instance, in 2020, the White House Office of Science and Technology Policy had issued a call to action for experts to build AI tools that can be applied to a new COVID-19 data set. Manually going through large data sets is cost and time prohibitive, so writing AI programs that can do the sifting allows researchers to get the most important components faster.

Organizational Context, Big Data, and the Ecological Fallacy

Everyone and everything exist with an environment and have a context specific to their surroundings. When an organization or system attempts to use big data to drive lower-level processes, results may vary from expectations or goals due not to the leadership or rollout process but to what is called an *ecological fallacy*. As opposed to an atomistic fallacy, this is a reasoning fallacy in the interpretation of statistical data where inferences about the nature of individuals are made from inferences about the group to which those individuals belong. This means that relationships between health care process performance measures (PPMs) and outcomes can differ in magnitude and even direction for patients (individual level) versus higher-level units (data are aggregated at higher levels, e.g., health care facilities and systems). Such differences can arise because organizational-level relationships ignore PPM outcome relationships for patients within organizations (Finney et al., 2011).

Organizations may have different *confounding variables* (variables that have an unintentional effect on the dependent variable) than at the individual level. If a patient-level PPM is related to better patient outcomes at the individual level, then that care process should be encouraged. However, research findings in a multilevel analysis (aggregated individual data up to the organizational level) have demonstrated that the proportion of patients receiving PPM care across facilities is linked to poor hospital outcomes.

Instead of stopping the patient-level PPM, the more appropriate suggestion might be finding interventions that foster the better outcomes at the organizational level (Finney et al., 2011). Interventions might include improving the work environment, using staff and patient satisfaction scores as a marker. In order to understand and use big data appropriately, remember that big data will always need to be contextualized in the environment, including social, economic, and political contexts (Graham, 2012).

The same ecological fallacies can happen with *performance measures* (PMs) in a health care system. PMs quantify the extent to which a process of care that has been shown to cause or predict positive outcomes among participants at an individual level in empirical studies is applied to patients in health care facilities (e.g., hospitals) (Cutler & McClellan, 2002001; Fonarow et al., 2007). PMs are implemented on the assumption that processes of care linked to positive patient-level outcomes in clinical trials and other research will be associated with positive facility-level outcomes when aggregated to the facility level. However, without using a multilevel analysis, outcomes for the same PM can show different relationships at different levels of analysis. These reasons include the following:

- Loss of information within higher-level units

- Different confounding variables at the patient and facility levels

- Effect modification (Finney et al., 2011)

Of course, when I say multilevel analysis, I am talking about statistical methods. Instead of making this a mini statistics course, the following is good example of what can happen. It is important to remember that a leader cannot choose to be ignorant about anything. While you might be thinking this is a lot about statistics and research, having an understanding about how others in your system may be applying data correctly or incorrectly has a direct effect on your practice! Do you really want to make a practice change if there is a chance that an ecological fallacy was made with the data? It is absolutely important to know about your data, as well as who and how people are aggregating data in an organization and the health care system!

The fact that higher-level data show less than the desired rates of improvement does not mean there is not a clinical significance at the individual patient level. It is important to understand that a smaller than desired rate of statistical significance does not mean that the clinical significance is less than desired too. Individual-level data must be reviewed as well with higher-level data, particularly through advanced

---

A CONSIDERATION FOR SYSTEMS THINKING

Early Understanding of the Ecological Fallacy

Discrepancies in relationships at different levels of analysis were most prominently brought to attention by social scientist William S. Robinson in 1950. Using 1930 US census data, he found that the state-level correlation between the percentage of foreign-born adult residents and the English-language illiteracy rate was −0.53. In other words, states with higher percentages of foreign-born residents had lower illiteracy rates (Robinson, 1950).

However, a closer look at the lower-level, individual-level data showed that the individual-level correlation (ignoring state of residence, which is a higher level) between foreign-born status and English illiteracy was positive (0.12). Foreign-born individuals were more likely to be illiterate in English. The unexpected negative correlation at the state level reflected the fact that foreign-born individuals had tended to settle in states where literacy rates among native-born citizens were higher (Robinson, 1950).

Had we looked only at the higher-level data, we might have misunderstood literacy rates. We might have assumed all the residents of a state noted for lower literacy rates had low literacy rates themselves when in fact native citizens had higher rates of literacy. By looking at both the higher-level and lower-level data, we have a different and more complete understanding of the issue.

The problem with inferring individual-level relationships from aggregated data was subsequently called the ecological fallacy.

multilevel or mixed-effects methods to better capture and understand PM–outcome relationships across and within health care facilities.

Your Role in Big Data

Corporate Leader

As the corporate leader, the individual in charge of chairing a team to standardize care, incorporating process measures, and ensuring goals are met, it is imperative that you understand big data and the positive and potentially negative effects it can have. If there is a lack of understanding or an improper interpretation, this can

---

A CONSIDERATION FOR SYSTEMS THINKING

Big Data and Performance Measures

One example of data aggregation issues was reviewed by researchers who examined National Quality Forum (NQF) performance measures for treating patients with acute myocardial infarction. They found that higher rates of provision of the practices recommended by the NQF were at best only slightly related to lower hospital-level, risk-adjusted 30-day mortality rates among patients with acute myocardial infarction from more than 900 hospitals. Further research (Werner & Bradlow, 2006) was conducted with a more comprehensive analysis of data from approximately 3,600 acute care hospitals. This research showed findings that facilities in the top and bottom quartiles in terms of proportion of patients receiving processes of care recommended by the Centers for Medicare & Medicaid Services for acute myocardial infarction, heart failure, and pneumonia differed only slightly in risk-adjusted 30-day and 1-year mortality rates. Weak relationships between clinical care quality and patient satisfaction were also noted at the facility and practice levels (Bradley et al., 2006).

Both studies (Bradley et al., 2006; Werner & Bradlow, 2006) pointed to a variety of factors that may have accounted for the weak facility-level associations, including potential facility-level confounding factors (e.g., patient safety processes). What was missed was that even though facility-level performance on these care processes was only weakly associated with aggregated facility outcomes, patients who did receive this type of care may have had significantly better outcomes than patients who did not when individual-level data are examined (Finney et al., 2011). If you are that patient who will benefit from the provision of a certain PM, you would want that treatment, right? Could you imagine being told that since the PM did not show statistically different improvements in care at an organizational or system level, you cannot receive the care? Sometimes we must provide care that is clinically significant but may not always be statistically significant.

have a negative effect on both patient outcomes at the facility and individual levels and on the leader in that facility who championed the performance measure. It is imperative that big data are analyzed by someone who knows how to perform multilevel analysis. Not every person with a statistical background and not every statistical software program can do this appropriately.

When data demonstrate less than stellar high-level results for PMs, you can help by taking a deeper dive into the data. Facility leaders will quite often say, we are different here, and to some extent, that is correct. Contextual factors at play with their patients can have significant effects on their outcomes. Not taking these factors into consideration can cause you to miss out on the opportunity to strengthen processes that will in turn improve patient outcomes.

Facility Leader

If you receive data only on facility-level PM–outcome relationships, you should view those relationships with caution. Although they may reflect PM–outcome relationships that were aggregated, these relationships may also differ in magnitude or even be in the opposite direction from patient-level relationships. With aggregated data, you can lose both the ability to estimate the direction and magnitude of bias and any ability to extend inferences reliably to less aggregated data. That is, the addition of more grouped data will not eliminate the bias (Piantadosi, 1994, p. 763).

Ideally, both patient-level and facility-level data would support the connection between PMs and outcomes. However, as a facility leader, there are things you must consider when reviewing your data at a unit, organization, or system level. Take the following thoughts about individual and aggregated data into consideration before changing care processes:

- Ideally, both patient-level and facility-level data (AKA: multilevel data) would support the connection between PMs and outcomes.

    - If patient-level PM-specific care demonstrates positive outcomes, this should be evidence to encourage and support continued clinical practice even if the outcome is negative or not statistically significant at the facility or higher levels.

    - Remember, provision of care should be prioritized to the individual patient (not individualized to the provider or facility).

    - Instances that demonstrate facilities in which PM performance is positively related to outcomes but is not as strong at the individual patient

level suggest looking at means of improving patient-level relationships
(PMs tailored to the patient).

When given facility-level and system-level outcomes on any measure, process,
performance, and even staff or patient satisfaction, understand your data and
how they were analyzed (Finney et al., 2011). A lot of this last section spoke to
clinical patient measures; however, this is just as applicable with patient satisfaction data, employee engagement scores, and financial and operational measures.
In order to be successful in leading in the system, you need to be able to see the
forest despite the trees and have individuals at each facility help you see the trees
despite the forest.

Successful Teams

As a corporate leader, you may be involved in leading teamwork, chairing multifa-
cility meetings, and ensuring goals and changes are met on time. In the last chapter,
we discussed components for successful teams, but there are a few more components
to consider if you are at a corporate level. Understanding the impact and contextual
factors that can be missing from your data as we just discussed, how can you bring
the local, individual facility context to meetings and champion goals?

Successfully Pulling Together Complex Teams

The guidelines mentioned in chapter 7 for choosing appropriate team members
also apply here, but there is an added complexity to building a systemwide team.
In a large system, how do you keep a team small enough to function while also
making it representative? Factors you should consider when deciding how many
and, more specifically, who should be on your team (Arnold, 2010) are tasks,
representation, diversity, skill levels, and development needs. These factors are
as follows:

- *Tasks:* What are you asking the team to do? Is it highly independent or interdependent work? Is there precedent in that it has been done before, or is it an entirely
  new task?

- *Representation:* Do you have a representative from each part of the system, process,
  or other stakeholder groups? Is there representation at the individual, facility, and
  system levels? Do you need representation at all three levels?

- *Diversity:* Do you have functional geographic, educational, and transdisciplinary diversity within the team? Do you have representatives who can wear multiple hats so that you can limit the number of people who need to be in the room while still representing everyone? If you have multiple critical access hospitals or multiple clinics, can one individual who works in one of these facilities represent the perspective instead of having one person from every site? Diversity also includes things such as different social and ethnic backgrounds, race, different genders, and sexual orientations.

- *Skill levels:* Do you have a good mix of people who have been on successful teams to help those who have not? These individuals tend to assimilate good team behaviors into whatever team they are on.

- *Developmental needs:* Are you asking the same people to every team? Many organizations continually ask the same dependable people to work on important teams. Perhaps you have gone to the well just a few too many times and need to invest in some new blood and fresh perspectives. This takes more effort on your part, but you run less risk of burning out individuals.

Depending on these factors, you may want to add or subtract a few folks from the mix.

A system- or corporate-level employee is someone who sees the forest despite the trees. It is imperative that facility- and individual-level employees help the system employee see the trees, as much as it is the responsibility of the corporate-level employee to help the facility-level employee to see the forest. Working together on

---

A CONSIDERATION FOR SYSTEMS THINKING

The Ringlemann Effect

At the turn of the twentieth century, a French agricultural engineer named Maximilian Ringlemann analyzed the pull force of people alone and in groups as they pulled on a rope. As Ringlemann added more and more people at the rope, he discovered that the total force generated by the group rose, but the average force exerted by each group member declined. The idea that a group team effort results in increased effort, therefore, is not always true.

Ringlemann attributed this lack of effort as "social loafing," where the effort of the group will disguise the fact that individuals are not pulling their weight (Arnold, 2010).

Creating the Patient Experience Brand across the Health Care System: It Takes Leadership

The health care system's well-established mission statement and values are the beginning of the patient experience journey. The mission statement clearly articulates how the organization—regardless of the number of entities or size—will meet the needs of patients and customers through engaged employees and medical staff. The values are the foundation guiding the behaviors of all who serve patients and their loved ones. Formally describing the patient experience initiative as a system priority and linking it to the mission and values is the critical first step in communicating to everyone how patients are to be treated. Next, the System Executive Team carefully chooses one of its own to serve as the Patient Experience Executive Sponsor. This person, who is influential, passionate about patient experience, and able to generate enthusiasm and excitement, believes it is important for everyone to consider the impact of each strategic, operational, and/or clinical decision or policy on patients' experiences.

The Executive Sponsor willingly and actively participates in key patient experience activities and meetings, including inviting patients who have recently received care at one or more of the system's entities to give reports and tell their stories at the health care system's Board of Directors (BOD) meetings. These stories told by real patients create another level of knowing that poignantly captures the human experience. Putting a face on the patient satisfaction metrics allows board members to ask pertinent questions of those served as well as of themselves as they deliberate the future of the health care system. Devoting time to patients and their experiences on BOD meeting agendas is a challenge given the plethora of competing priorities; however, it clearly demonstrates the level of organizational commitment to patients' experiences with their care.

Creating the infrastructure to support the patient experience initiative is the vital next step. A Chief Patient Experience Officer with a well-defined Patient Experience (PEX) department operationalizes the strategic initiative for the organization. The PEX department must be given the same stature as any other critical function in the organization (e.g., Finance, Patient Safety or Quality). The Chief Patient Experience Officer brings formal and informal leaders together from across the system. These leaders own the plan, establish milestones, chair facility-level Patient Experience Committees, and create the accountability framework all employees and medical staff within each and every facility are held. Evidence-based interventions to improve patients' experiences are selected at three levels: (1) system level to address improvement opportunities present at the majority of facilities, (2) facility level to address one or two

(continued)

additional improvement opportunities unique to the facility, and (3) unit or department level to address an additional improvement opportunity or two that have not been identified at the levels above. In this way, the system moves forward in a clearly defined manner that will surely bring success as quarterly results are reviewed.

Amy Steinbinder, PhD, RN, NE-BC

teams, whether facility level or system level, requires great communication and collaboration.

Key Points

- The goal of a system or corporate employee is not to make all the decisions that trickled down but to be the support person.

- Managing relationships across organizations is a tough job.

- Organizations form or become part of another system because they believe there is some value in the relationship that has a positive outcome.

- Ensuring great communication and collaboration can offset concerns of a merger or acquisition and over time will build trust and a brand in the community.

- An atomistic fallacy can occur when one makes inferences about groups or aggregates from individuals or individual-level data.

- "Big data" is the term for a collection of large and complex data sets that are considered difficult to process using run-of-the-mill database management tools.

- The ecological fallacy in the interpretation of statistical data occurs when inferences about the nature of individuals are deduced from inferences about the group to which those individuals belong.

CHAPTER 9

Moving Everyone Forward

Without reflection, we go blindly on our way,
creating more unintended consequences, and
failing to achieve anything useful.

—Margaret Wheatley

The whole is only as strong as its weakest link. It is important that every department, unit, facility, and organization work together to provide seamless care along the care continuum in a system. In the previous few chapters, we discussed collaboration, communication, teams, and data for both the facility and corporate levels. This chapter will focus on how to move the whole organization forward through strategic thinking, planning, and unity.

Being One in a System through Joint Goals

Moving the organization forward involves having united goals, the same language, a mission, and a vision. Strategic planning is an organization's process of defining its strategy or direction and making decisions on allocating its resources to pursue this strategy. To determine the future direction of the organization, it is necessary to understand its current position and the possible avenues through which it can pursue particular courses of action.

Typically, the process of creating joint goals is done through strategic planning at the board and executive levels. It is very important that the board and executives during the planning session do not get into the operational detail. This is for the staff to decide. If the board gets into operational detail, they are not being strategic. And of course, employees should inform the strategic plan. However, their role is to determine how to operationalize and produce the expected outcomes.

Depending on the maturity of the health care system, strategic planning may include more managers and direct-care providers. Even if you are not involved in strategic planning, to lead in the system, you need to be a strategic thinker! However, best practice would be to include all employees in some level of involvement in the strategic planning process.

A strategic plan should not be something that only lives on the intranet site or in a fancy organizational poster. Nor is it something that gets attention only when preparing for a quarterly board meeting.

If strategic thinking can lead to redefined core strategies or changes in the health care industry, what does the future of care look like, and who envisions that? Think about the Patient Protection and Affordable Care Act (PPACA), specifically accountable care organizations (ACOs) and the focus on prevention and care across the continuum. Now, that is not something new but rather something many have been advocating as a flip in the system. The idea is to focus on primary care in the community with patients getting care in a hospital only after other options are exhausted or if there is no better setting for the care needed. How do we take the law and think and plan strategically for this future starting with nurses? The strategic plan of an organization is not the only driver of strategy.

A CONSIDERATION FOR SYSTEMS THINKING	
Best practices on including frontline staff in strategic planning:	• Provide regular updates at staff meetings.
• Provide opportunities for feedback when planning.	• Explain the why behind the goals.
• Seek input from employees when determining how to operationalize the plan.	• Connect the dots: Demonstrate how each employee impacts the plan.

A Strategy within a Strategy: Nurse Care Management in a BPCIA Model

Bundled Payment for Care Improvement Advanced (BPICA) was developed by the Center for Medicare & Medicaid Innovation as part of the Affordable Care Act, to test innovative payment and service delivery models that have the potential to reduce governmental payers' expenditures while preserving or enhancing the quality of care for their beneficiaries (Centers for Medicare & Medicaid Services [CMS], 2019). The goal of the program is care delivery innovation and redesign to optimize patient outcomes in a value-based setting, tying outcomes to payment. This means that certain Diagnostic Related Groups (DRGs) moved from being paid fee-for-service to a retrospective bundled payment starting at the anchor inpatient admission to the hospital, plus the postacute care and all related services up to 90 days after hospital discharge (CMS, 2019). Having years of experience leading out the BPCIA program, here are some of my key takeaways for a successful program.

RN Model of care

The foundation of building an RN model of care for a BPCIA program includes working at the top of your RN license and must begin by reviewing the ANA standard of practice and nursing independent scope of practice. The idea of operating at the top of your license means practicing to the full extent of your education and training instead of spending time doing something that could be done by a different role (Virkstis, 2014). The program also needs to include RN electronic tools, standard work, and structures to manage practice and process by reducing waste in the system. With this program having such a financial impact on the organization, several stakeholders providing "directives" to the BPCIA nurses can cause several difficulties: (1) the stakeholders are not nurses, (2) the stakeholders are not familiar with an RN's independent scope of practice, and (3) the meaning of the program to improve the quality of care and outcomes for patients can be lost in the financial pressure.

In the BPCIA, the organization has fiscal responsibility for all of the patients' care for 90 days. If the RN Care Managers are unsuccessful at providing proactive care coordination, it could potentially have a significant financial impact on the organization and, most important, the patient's quality of care. This, in turn, can affect quality scores, the reputation of the organization, and perhaps loss of business. What can be detrimental to the program is when different stakeholders create pathways to reduce the financial risk without creating a patient-centered approach. This quote was meaningful to me: "They focused all their resources on the one best way: they reduced slack to be lean and mean, and they reduced redundancy to ensure everyone and everything was focused on their strategic priorities. As a result, they lost peripheral vision and perspective" (Westley et al., 2007, p. 67).

(continued)

Patient-centered quality of care includes nurses operating within their independent scope of practice, being able to develop patient-centered care plans, building a patient–RN therapeutic relationship, and assessing the patient's social determinants of health, within an evidence-based clinical care pathway. Key foundation components include standard work for each discipline, clinical decision trees, escalation pathways for when patients are off track, and foundational care management education. These patient-centered care plans are built on key nursing knowledge of motivational interviewing, stages of change, patient education assessments, teach-back methods, and so on. Patient engagement is an increasingly important component strategy to reform health care by patient activation, and patients who become more engaged have better outcomes and care experiences (Hibbard & Greene, 2013).

The root of value-based care is providing the highest level of patient-centered quality of care. In theory, the highest quality of care will decrease health care costs and produce a return on investment. Emerging evidence indicates that interventions that tailor support to the individuals' level of activation and that build skills and confidence are effective in increasing patient activation, although there is limited evidence on the impact on costs (Hibbard & Greene, 2013). Providing the BPCIA nurses with continuing care management education will be important for them to understand managing

length of stay, patient utilization, CMS rules and regulations, and postacute levels of care and requirements to prevent avoidable utilization postdischarge. One strategy to enhance professional case management education with positive learning outcomes is to incorporate interactive lectures and small group case study discussions (Liu et al., 2009).

Building a value-based care program includes having standard work to provide the nurses with tools to perform their work; it allows better management of the practice and reduces waste in the system. Creating standard work is about efficiency, accuracy, and safety, allowing clinicians to create, test, and improve their work (Quisenberry, 2021). Best practice in supporting a collaborative learning environment is to foster a shared governance model and include the nurse in creating their standard work. This will ensure accuracy of the work being performed and create buy-in from the nurses on the process of creating their standard work while increasing engagement and staff satisfaction. Recognizing that creativity is good for employees' engagement and skill building, having the nurse develop the process will enhance their confidence in the process and allow them to master their jobs and grow their understanding of new aspects of their work every day (Quisenberry, 2021).

Our goal is to provide comprehensive patient-centered care coordination to optimize patients' health with innovative strategies to improve quality, safety, and health care utilization. Creating a

(continued)

vision and scope of work for the nurses will include Rundio's (2016) ACO reimbursement model of an umbrella. The sphere of the umbrella is all of the services the patient can receive: Medical home, primary care, acute care, psychological/mental health care, rehabilitative care, outpatient care, and home care are grouped under the horizontal bundled billing (Rundio, 2016). The handle of the umbrella is the quality of care. The nurses need to envision holding the quality-of-care handle, supporting the patient under their umbrella to receive the best care and outcomes.

The nurse education plan for nurses new to this type of program can include a mix of lectures and shadowing of different nursing roles where the nurses have identified areas of opportunity such as in-home health or clinic. In creating a value-based transitional care role, start where the patient begins in the process. For elective bundles patients, this begins when the patient is being assessed for surgery. Having the nurse do a thorough assessment on the patient's current living environment, support systems, social determinants of health, and current medical optimization needed for the patient will ensure a smoother and shorter anchor admission stay because the patient will be properly prepared for postacute care and needs prior to the surgery. The nurses need education on care management, motivational interviewing, independent scope of practice, trauma-informed care, social determinants of health, and building patient-centered care plans. The lecture

portions will be with experts on the topics followed by shadow experiences with the inpatient RN Case Managers, Transitional Care Nurses, and our ambulatory RN Care Managers. This will support the nurses in creating their social network and making connections to support their work through network weaving.

Once they have completed their education training, the nurses should use evidence-based guidelines to identify tools they can use to fill in the gaps of care—for example, creating pathways and tools for readmission risk assessment, patient education teach-back tools, follow-up phone call scripts, and escalation pathways if their patients are at risk. Confirmation audits of using the tools, barrier trackers, and data should be incorporated into your daily management system for continuous process improvement. Key follow-through activities for microsystem leaders are following fundamentals of improvement, creating a data wall to display ongoing performance measures, creating and updating our playbook, and maintaining the storyboard of our improvement journey (Nelson et al., 2007). Measures to track success are important. Two such measured that were used when auditing the program were tracking the confidence of the nurses in the care they provided as well as measuring the perceived helpfulness of the care management processes and tools that were created to improve care. Utilizing a barrier tracker will help you determine your next emerging cycle and support an appreciative learning culture.

(continued)

Attributes of a Strategic Thinker

Many individuals who are involved in strategic thinking usually do not have any formal, informal, or continued education to inform their planning. There are many books and consultants who can help with this, but what are some of the major attributes or competencies of strategic thinking? Five attributes or competencies that can help you become a better strategic thinker are as follows:

1. Strategic thinkers have a *systems perspective*, which means they are able to understand implications of any action from start to end and see how they impact the system as a whole and the individual providing direct patient care. They can interpolate as well as extrapolate information and how that impacts the organization.

2. Strategic thinkers are *intent focused*, which means they are more determined to succeed at the mission and are not as distracted by less pertinent issues in the environment. They place appropriate energy and attention as long as needed to achieve the goal and are not distracted by the latest trend or fad.

3. They can think *in time*, which means they are able to keep in mind the past, present, and future in order to make the needed changes. This is not about letting past failures dictate what should or should not be done in the future but about lessons learned. Remember, a good idea at the wrong time is a bad idea.

4. They are *hypothesis driven*, ensuring that both creative and critical thinking are incorporated into strategy making. Understanding what the literature shows and what innovators and futurists say, as well as making your own connections about what will be next, helps to drive that innovation, which may not always succeed, but you still need a hypothesis before you can do anything!

5. They are *intelligent opportunists*, meaning that they are responsive to good opportunities. While we mentioned not getting sidetracked by trends earlier, there are still opportunities that exist today and did not exist at the time the strategic plan was created! Does that mean we ignore everything and forge forward with blinders? No. Use your intelligence to decide which opportunities are worth picking up along the way (Liedtka, 1998).

The implication for health care systems, organizations, and executives and managers is that they must find ways to identify and cultivate future leaders with the capacity to think strategically. There is the question, is a leader born or made? Both nature and nurture are important, but now that you are on this earth, there is not much you can do on the nature side. With that said, what can you nurture to grow the abilities you do have? Some approaches to develop your strategic-thinking ability include the following:

- **Immersion:** Immersion is important because people need significant "soak time" in an environment to build powerful mental models. As was noted in a prior chapter, in relationship to talent mapping, you cannot necessarily move leaders around quickly without potential negative effects. Moving people too rapidly from area to area or position to position does not allow time to master the core dynamics of each new situation.

A CONSIDERATION FOR SYSTEMS THINKING

Strategic Thinking versus Strategic Planning

To think strategically is to seek innovation and imagine new and very different futures that may lead the system to redefine its core strategies and even its industry. Strategic planning's role is to realize and to support strategies developed through the strategic thinking process and to integrate these back into the business (Graetz, 2002).

- *Apprenticeships:* One of the best ways to learn to think strategically is to work closely with experts in these areas. Typically, nursing tends to have mentor or preceptor relationships. You can have more than one mentor. I have chosen different mentors, each with a strength I admire and want to build in myself. A mentorship provides those who are not experts with the opportunity to observe and learn from experts. And, mentors can change over time, and that is okay!

- *Simulations:* Simulation rotations have been a great tool in clinical practice but can also be used by others to enhance learning activities. Just like a simulated code, you can practice, fail safely, and try again.

- *Case-based education:* You can develop your strategic thinking by exposing yourself to a diverse range of realistic "cases" and letting yourself reflect on the experiences so you can absorb the lessons.

- *Cognitive reshaping:* Sometimes, you need to just think differently, which is a tough thing to do. Completing mental exercises helps to create new mental habits. An example of a mental exercise is the "go to the balcony" exercise, where you step back from what is going on and try to get a different perspective of the situation. This is helpful in tense and difficult meetings. Once you get a unique perspective, you can adjust strategies accordingly (Watkins, 2007).

Once a strategic plan is created for the system, it is usually rolled out to individual facilities and departments. From there, the plan is operationalized, which includes answering the question, "How are we going to accomplish these goals?" Start with ensuring your staff are involved in deciding how to get the work done. Shared leadership/governance is a great structure for operationalizing the strategic plan on a unit or department level. Then, focus on a communication plan so that everyone knows which direction they are supposed to go! Methods to help communicate a strategic plan are

- Printing and handing it out at staff meetings

- Having the facility executives and nursing executives hold forums to share their visions

- Working with unit and department shared leadership to share and disseminate their plan and how to operationalize it

- Placing it on posters and posting it in every major employee area and on your organization's intranet

- Incorporating your strategic plan into the orientation process for new employees

- Emailing regular updates

In addition to the system strategic plan, nursing may have created a strategic plan in Magnet-designated facilities that further demonstrates the interwoven nature of nursing as an integral part of the system strategic plan. This nursing strategic plan should be communicated widely to nursing and other disciplines.

Supporting Components in the System

No system is just a conglomerate of organizations. Many components help to pull everyone together. These components include support departments, standardized policies, procedures, languages, and forms. Each of these components helps to facilitate collaboration and communication among all the units and organizations in a system.

Support Departments

Incorporating support departments is important in leading the system forward. Even if a department does not have nurses, sharing the nursing strategic plan and communicating the work to be done enable others to understand their potential scope of work as well. Nurses in a system or organization may defer to a support department for its expertise in operationalizing the strategic plan but take the advice as if it is the final word. These departments may include the legal, risk, and information technology (IT) departments. When issues arise or controversy exists, these departments have expertise in the areas of legal, risk, human resources, and IT (to name a few), but they do not have expertise in nursing scope of practice or professional standards.

As the nurse leading in the system, you are an equal part of the system, bringing invaluable knowledge to the table. No one can represent or guide nursing practice but a nurse. You cannot defer your responsibility to someone who is not a nurse. As you partner with various support departments, to be successful, watch how you frame your questions and scope of work with them. This will impact the way they respond to you and how they may or may not try to control your area of expertise.

Remember, one component in many support departments is to decrease risk to the organization, whether risk to employees, risk to electronic information, risk to patients, or legal risk to the organization. These departments will want to decrease risk brought about by nursing practice as well and play on the safe side of practice. Innovation is not easily done if we are always doing things by the rules. When you are working with various support departments, ask them to come with you on a journey. Tell them that you want to do something and need their help to do it as safely as possible. You are not asking them for permission. I know in some organizations, this may seem like heresy, but remember, as the nurse leader, you are the expert in nursing and nursing practice. You may have to work a while to create partnerships with individuals to have success in collaboration.

Standard Language

Speaking the same language in your system is important. If each organization has a different definition for things, your ability to function well will decrease. Too much time will be spent reconciling definitions before work can even start, or even worse, work starts, but it becomes clear during the process that teamwork needs to halt to get everyone on the same page with definitions! In the appendix at the end of this book is a starter list of some key terms and words that should be standardized.

A CONSIDERATION FOR SYSTEMS THINKING

What Is Human Factors Engineering?

Human factors engineering is the science dealing with the application of information on physical and psychological characteristics to the design of devices and systems for human use. It may seem like overkill to have a specialist design a standard template like a policy or procedure, but they have the knowledge and expertise to design it in such a way that it improves compliance and understanding while decreasing errors. If you are going to standardize a form or template (including electronic forms), using a human factors engineer should be considered.

Standard Forms

Now that you are standardizing your language, time to standardize forms!

I can hear you, where is the personalization? You do not need it. Does it add value? Does it improve patient care? Or does it slow the process down for others? Learn to pick your battles. Learn when to be collaborative and come to consensus on lower-level items like form design. Better yet, have someone with a human factors background help design templates for your forms, including policies, procedures, and team charters.

Charters

While we are talking about standardization and forms, charters are necessary for any team but are particularly important in a complex organization or system. A charter document that is developed in a group setting clarifies team direction while establishing boundaries. It is developed early during the formation of the team. The charter should be developed in a group session to encourage understanding and buy-in. A team charter should include the following sections:

- *Team purpose:* The purpose drives the deliverables and your SMART (Specific, Measurable, Achievable, Relevant, and Time-bound) goal(s). If you are not clear, then you run the risk of missing the mark with your deliverables.

- *Duration and time commitment:* The amount of time the team will be working together needs to be documented (e.g., deliverables will be done in six months) as well as the frequency of meetings (such as once a week or monthly).

- *Scope (in scope/out of scope):* Thinking through the scope helps to define the beginning and end of the spectrum and helps the team chair identify things that are outside of the scope, minimizing scope creep.

- *Members:* Chair, co-chair (if needed), and members should be listed individually. Ad hoc members also can be listed (those who might be needed for specialty advice along the way but not at each meeting). The sponsor (usually the executive in to which the chair reports) needs to be assigned and listed.

- *Deliverable(s):* This provides an opportunity to begin with the end in mind. This is where the sponsor can establish or oversee goal development. Goals should take on a SMART format.

- *Reporting plan:* This defines how the team will communicate progress to the sponsor.

A sample charter is included in the appendix of this book.

Standard Policies and Procedures

We did touch on the reason to standardize in prior chapters, but what is important about standardizing policies and procedures is to have a policy on policies. I am not a fan of policies and therefore try to remove as many from existence as possible. However, there is still a need for some. What usually gets in the way of standardizing policies and procedures across vastly different health care settings and organizations is the lack of a policy that helps people understand the ins and outs of policies in their system.

A policy on policy is also a great way to set the tone for Evidence Based Practice (EBP) in your system. As mentioned earlier, appropriate standardization is needed to push an organization into good outcomes for patients. Remember that EBP occurs when the clinicians contextualize the best available research evidence by integrating it with their clinical judgment and the patient's values and expectations. No one clinician can know all the evidence, let alone keep up with it all. Thus, the best evidence must be placed in policies, procedures, clinical pathways, standards of

---

A CONSIDERATION FOR SYSTEMS THINKING

When is it a policy, and when should it be a standard of care?

Why do I want to rid of the world of policies? Because once written, if someone does not follow it to a proverbial "T," then a clinician or, mainly, an organization can be cited by an accrediting body for "not following policy." My issue is that clinicians, such as nurses and advance practice nurses, are knowledge workers. A policy must be followed exactly, step by step, whereas a standard of care is a guideline. One may argue a policy does not need to be followed step by step, but accrediting organizations

like The Joint Commission will tell you otherwise. So, why not follow a policy step by step if it is evidence based? Remember EBP? EBP is patient preference, best evidence, and clinician judgment. A policy is full of the best evidence. But a policy cannot be written in such a way that would allow for clinician judgment or deviation. That is why standards of care exist. They provide the best evidence and then allow the nurse to use clinical judgment and patient preference to make the best decision.

What policies are in your organization that should be standards of care?

care, and the like. But how many times have these things been written with no evidence, let alone any evidence from peer-reviewed journals from the past five to six years?

I remember in 2010 trying to find evidence for fecal transplants. The "newest" evidence I could find was from the 1970s! Fast forward, there is more recent evidence. The review period for your policies, whether every year or every three years, should include an update to the literature when it exists, to support a practice to continue or to change.

Things to consider when writing your policy on policies:

- There will be method(s) of evidence grading that will be used across all the organizations and all disciplines.

- All policies will have facility input whether written by a volunteer group/person or an existing committee.

- Preapproval is required to develop a new policy or update a policy (stops people from different organizations updating something at will without a system effort).

- A written education plan should go hand in hand with the draft policy and will be refined as needed.

- Regulatory requirements are incorporated into policies and procedures.

- When there is contradictory evidence, move to using guidelines.

- Standards of practice exist for all professions. Nursing has standards of practice and therefore you do not need a policy for everything a nurse does. You will run the risk of getting your organization in trouble trying to maintain and practice to the standards of every word that was written into a well-meaning policy!

While there are preferred methods by discipline for grading and assessing evidence, it is important that we speak a common language not only across the system but across disciplines. As care continues to strengthen across the continuum, and care transitions and coordination become even more important, we all will be working in a much more interdisciplinary way.

If we work on interdisciplinary care guidelines, using different methods to evaluate the literature can slow progress of work. Having an interdisciplinary group decide on the one or two approaches to grading literature for the entire system will accelerate the ability to change and innovate care.

Excellence in Patient Care

As leaders in the system, the main reason we do anything is so that patients get the best care possible. No one gets up in the morning and thinks, *I am going to do what I can to stop patients from getting the best care.* What does happen is that our systems, structures, and personal biases prevent us from moving each part of the system forward, passively or actively. What are you doing today that is preventing the best of patient care from occurring?

A CONSIDERATION FOR SYSTEMS THINKING

Seven Reasons to Work in a Health Care System

1. You learn an awful lot. You get to see the good, the bad, and the ugly of different organizations. You see lots of very good ideas and some not so good ideas and how an organization reacts to both.

2. You get to work with many clever people. There are a lot of people in a health care system, so this is a great place to find at least one mentor for yourself.

3. You become part of a large community. While you will never know everyone, you will be a part of a community that many people are proud to belong to. Even after you leave, you will take many friendships and memories of the good with you.

4. They have lots of benefits. With health care changes, there are fewer perks than even a few years ago, but systems tend to have purchasing power and are able to provide better leverage in employee benefits and perks than smaller or single organizations.

5. You learn the art of politics. A multi-level health care system provides plenty of opportunities to acquire diplomacy and political skills. Once you leave the company (if you ever do), you will be able to use these skills no matter what you do or where you go.

6. You have time to reflect. At a small organization, change can happen much more quickly. Large organizations or systems do not move and cannot move at such a reckless pace, so you have time to learn and reflect.

7. You get a baseline, then you go and try to do it better. What do you think you can change? Make a list and see how many ambitions you can stick to or whether you finally succumb and realize that you do need the entire system to make things work (adapted from Stephens, 2010).

Key Points

- Moving the organization forward involves having joint goals, the same language, a mission, and a vision.

- Health care systems, organizations, executives, and managers must find ways to identify and cultivate future leaders with the capacity to think strategically.

- Once a strategic plan is created for the system, it is usually rolled out to individual facilities and departments. Allow the staff seats at the table to determine how it should be operationalized.

- No one can represent or guide nursing practice except a nurse.

Sample Components for System Support

As discussed in chapter 9, some system components support and facilitate collaboration and communication among constituent units and organizations. This appendix shows some examples.

Standard Language: Some Guidelines

Key Content

- **Key terms:** Any term that you think is unique to a policy or procedure that may need defining to understand the policy.

- **Acronyms:** While these do not need to be defined, it is advisable to write out the entire word the first time it is used and place the acronym in parentheses next to the word. Use initial capital letters as the term would appear if used in mid-sentence or mid-phrase. Capitalize only if it is a proprietary term, formal noun, program name, and so on.

  - Example: magnetic resonance imaging (MRI)

- Exception: Acronyms that have a standard, nontechnical meaning (RN, MD) do not need to be written out.

Key Considerations

- What do regulatory/accrediting bodies state about a term or definition?

- What does your legal and/or compliance department state about a definition? Remember, they are a resource; they should not be solely defining professional terms or terms that have an impact on a profession.

Some Writing Guidelines

- The definition does not need to be a complete sentence.

- Keep an entry as short as possible without sacrificing clarity. Occasionally, a second or phrase or sentence could be used to clarify a word or term used in the opening phrase or sentence. See entries below: *continuity of care; determinants of health; care coordination.*

- Do not restate the word or term in the definition.

- When in doubt, create the entry as a noun rather than a verb (e.g., "allocation" instead of "allocate").

Some Sample Terms and Definitions

- ***Care plans:*** A written communication that describes the care continuum for a defined patient or patient population. Individualization should be included with standards of care based on evidence. Plans should be interdisciplinary.

- ***Innovation:*** Can be a radical or brand-new idea or concept, as well as a recombining of current and disparate ideas that result in something new. It can also be something that is used in a new way!

- ***Nurse manager:*** A registered nurse with 24-hour/7-day accountability and responsibility for the overall supervision of employees and/or patient care.

- ***Order set:*** Preprinted or electronic set of orders subject to approval by the provider. These are provider initiated.

- *Policy:* A plan or course of action to help guide decision-making. Policies will be consistent with applicable federal and state laws and any accrediting agencies as well as professional standards. Such overarching statements should not go into unit- or facility-specific operational detail.

- *Preprinted orders:* Facility-approved form for a specific type of order that may or may not provide the ordering provider with options. These require authentication by the ordering provider before initiation by any clinician.

  - *Procedure (or process):* A series of specific tasks or actions designed to achieve a specific result. Should be separate from a policy. Procedures should not be embedded inside a policy but connected electronically with hyperlinks.

  - *Protocols:* Processes that generally include branch points (if/then statements), which can be objective or subjective (requiring judgment) that describe the steps to be taken during a care process.

  - *Standing orders:* Orders approved by the medical executive committee (MEC) that may be executed by the appropriate clinician prior to obtaining the individual provider order (either written or verbal). Limited to a subset of orders regarding a specific patient condition or circumstance in which necessary interventions are in order to provide timely and efficient care during a serious patient condition situation prior to obtaining a provider's verbal or written order.

  - *Team:* A small number of employees (5–10) with complementary skills who are committed to a common purpose, performance goals, and approach for which they are mutually accountable and responsible.

Some Health Care Practice Terms

- *Clinical practices:* A spectrum of care that can be delivered to a group of patients with a specific clinical condition. Based on the strength of the evidence.

- *Clinical practices—expected:* Based on the highest level of evidence-based research or strong consensus among providers and clinicians. Exceptions should be rare and justified through clinician or provider judgment and/or patient preferences.

- *Clinical practices—recommended:* Based on a high level of evidence, but with incomplete consensus among providers or clinicians. Exceptions are made based on the clinician's or provider's clinical judgment and patient preferences and can be either system-wide or facility specific.

- ***Nursing practice standards:*** Description of a competent level of nursing care as demonstrated by the critical thinking model known as the nursing process. The nursing process includes the components of assessment, diagnosis, outcomes identification, planning, implementation, and evaluation. The nursing process encompasses all significant actions taken by registered nurses and forms the foundation of the nurse's decision-making (ANA, 2021).

Sample Personal Development Form

	Personal Development Form
Date:	

Name:	
Mentor:	
Preceptor:	

Update Occurrence		
☐ Monthly	☐ Quarterly	☐ Other ( )

Reporting Details

Personal Mission Statement:

Three Short Term Goals (less than 1 year), Progress, and Timeframe:

Three Long Term Goals (1 year and beyond), Progress, and Timeframe:

Personal Development Needs to Achieve Goals:

Support/Education/Resources Needed:

Sample Team Charter

TEAM CHARTER		
Team Type: System_____ Organization_____ Unit_____		
Date: _____ Team Leader: _____		
Team Name		
Membership		
Executive Sponsor : _____		
Team Facilitator (if using one) : _____		
Team Members _____		
Role and Facility _____		
Scope ☐ Unit ☐ System ☐ Regional ☐ Service Line ☐ Organization/Facility		
Purpose for Team and End point for Team Meetings The objectives for this teams include: 1. 2. 3. 4. 5.		
Items out of Scope for Team: _____ Type of Meeting: In person_____ Conference Call_____ Video Conference_____ Meeting Frequency: _____ Time Keeper:_____		

	Deliverables/Tasks	Due Dates
1		
2		
3		
4		
5		

References

Agency for Healthcare Research and Quality (AHRQ). (2014). *About the National Quality Strategy*. http://www.ahrq.gov/workingforquality/about.htm

Agency for Healthcare Research and Quality (AHRQ). (2019). AHRQ's Core Competencies. Content last reviewed September 2019. https://www.ahrq.gov/cpi/corecompetencies /index.htm

Agency for Healthcare Research and Quality (AHRQ). (2022). Mission and budget. https:// www.ahrq.gov/cpi/about/mission/index.html

Agency for Healthcare Research and Quality (AHRQ). (2023a). Defining health systems. https://www.ahrq.gov/chsp/defining-health-systems/index.html

Agency for Healthcare Research and Quality (AHRQ). (2023b). Evidence-based Practice Center (EPC) reports. https://www.ahrq.gov/research/findings/evidence-based-reports /index.html

American Nurses Association. (2010). Nursing's social policy statement: The essence of the profession. American Nurses Association.

American Nurses Association. (2015). *Guide to the code of ethics for nurses with interpretive statements: Development, interpretation, and application* (2nd ed.). American Nurses Association.

American Nurses Association. (2021). *Nursing: Scope and standards of practice* (4th ed.). American Nurses Association.

APRN Consensus Work Group & the National Council of State Boards of Nursing APRN Advisory Committee. (2008, July 7). *Consensus model for APRN regulation: Licensure, accreditation, certification & education.* APRN Joint Dialogue Group Report. chrome -extension://efaidnbmnnnibpcajpcglclefindmkaj/https://www.ncsbn.org/public-files /Consensus_Model_for_APRN_Regulation_July_2008.pdf

Arnold, K. (2010, December 3). The optimal team size is. . . . [Blog post]. http://www .extraordinaryteam.com/optimal-team-size/

Aykac, A. (2013). Jack Welch & Jeff R. Immelt: Leadership styles [Presentation slides]. http://www.slideshare.net/alperay/jack-welch-and-jeff-immelt

Baker, L., Birnbaum, H., Geppert, J., Mishol, D., & Moyneur, E. (2003). The relationship between technology availability and health care spending. *Health Affairs, 22*(Suppl. 1), 537–551. https://doi.org/10.1377/hlthaff.w3.537

Bauer, M. S., & Kirchner, J. (2020). Implementation science: What is it and why should I care? *Psychiatry Research, 283,* 112376.

Big Data Senior Steering Group. (2016). *The federal big data research and development strategic plan.* http://digitalcommons.unl.edu/scholcom/20

Boamah, S. A., Laschinger, H. K. S., Wong, C., & Clarke, S. (2018). Effect of transformational leadership on job satisfaction and patient safety outcomes. *Nursing Outlook, 66*(2), 180–189.

Boyd, D. (2010, April 29). *Privacy and publicity in the context of big data.* Address at the WWW 2010 Conference, Raleigh, NC. http://www.danah.org/papers/talks/2010 /WWW2010.html

Bradley, E. H., Herrin, J., Elbel B., McNamara, R., Magid, D., Nallamothu, B., Wang, Y., Normand, S-L. T., Spertus, J. A., & Krumholz, H. (2006). Hospital quality for acute myocardial infarction: Correlations among process measures and relationship with short-term mortality. *Journal of the American Medical Association, 296,* 72–78.

The Budget and Economic Outlook Fiscal Years 2022 to 2032, US Congressional Budget Office. (2022, May). U.S.—defense outlays and forecast as a percentage of GDP 2032. *Statista.*

Burns, J. M. (1978). *Leadership.* Harper & Row.

Cahan, E. M., Kocher, R., & Bohn, R. (2020). Why isn't innovation helping reduce health care costs. *Health Affairs Blog.*

Carucci, R. (2017, November 13). Executives fail to execute strategy because they're too internally focused. *Harvard Business Review.* https://hbr.org/2017/11/executives-fail-to -execute-strategy-because-theyre-too-internally-focused

Caza, A., Caza, B. B., & Posner, B. Z. (2021). Transformational leadership across cultures: Follower perception and satisfaction. *Administrative Sciences, 11*(1), 32.

Centers for Disease Control, National Center for Health Statistics. (2022). Health expenditures. https://www.cdc.gov/nchs/fastats/health-expenditures.htm

Centers for Medicare & Medicaid Services. (2012). Shared Savings Program. https://www.cms.gov/medicare/medicare-fee-for-service-payment/sharedsavingsprogram

Centers for Medicare & Medicaid Services. (2019). Bundled Payments for Care Improvement (BPCI) initiative: General information. https://innovation.cms.gov/initiatives/bundled-payments

Centers for Medicare & Medicaid Services. (2022a). What is an ACO? https://innovation.cms.gov/innovation-models/aco

Center for Medicare & Medicaid Services (2022b). National coverage. https://innovation.cms.gov/innovation-models/aco

Chalmers, I., & Glasziou, P. (2009). Avoidable waste in the production and reporting of research evidence. *The Lancet, 374*(9683), 86–89. https://doi.org/10.1016/S0140-6736(09)60329-9

Chesbrough, H., & Garman, A. (2009, December). How open innovation can help you cope in lean times. *Harvard Business Review, 87*(12), 68–76.

Chow, M., Hendrick, A., Skierczynski, B. A., & Zhenqiang, L. (2008). A 36-hospital time and motion study: How do medical-surgical nurses spend their time? *The Permanente Journal, 12*(3), 25–34. https://doi.org/10.7812/tpp/08-021

Collins, J. (2001). *Good to great: Why some companies make the leap and others don't.* Harper Collins.

Covey, S. (2004). *The 7 habits of highly effective people: Powerful lessons in personal change.* Free Press.

Cutler, D. M., & McClellan, M. (2001). Is technological change in medicine worth it? *Health Affairs, 20,* 11–29.

Dawson, A. (2020). A practical guide to performance improvement: Change acceleration process and techniques to maintain improvements. *AORN Journal, 111*(1), 97–102.

Denning, S. (2010, November 17). The death—and reinvention—of management: Part 1 [Blog post]. http://stevedenning.typepad.com/steve_denning/2010/11/the-deathand-reinventionof-management-a-draft-synthesis.html

Denning, S. (2011, July 8). The five big surprises of radical management. *Forbes.* http://www.forbes.com/sites/stevedenning/2011/07/08/the-five-big-surprises-of-radical-management/

Department of Health and Human Services. (2023). About HHS. https://www.hhs.gov/about/index.html

Diez Roux, A.V. (2002). Theory and methods: A glossary for multilevel analysis. *Journal of Epidemiology & Community Health, 56,* 588–594. http://dx.doi.org/10.1136/jech.56.8.588

Donabedian, A. (1988). The quality of care: How can it be assessed? *Journal of the American Medical Association, 260*(12), 1743–1748.

Draper, S. W. (2013). *The Hawthorne, Pygmalion, placebo and other expectancy effects: Some notes.* Department of Psychology, University of Glasgow. http://www.psy.gla.ac.uk/~steve/hawth.html

Drucker, P. (1986). *The frontiers of management.* Harper & Row.

References

Federal Trade Commission, Antitrust Division of the Department of Justice. (2011). Statement of Antitrust Enforcement Policy regarding accountable care organizations participating in the Medicare Shared Savings Program. https://www.justice.gov/sites /default/files/atr/legacy/2011/10/20/276458.pdf

Finney, J. W., Humphreys, K., Kivlahan, D. R., & Harris, A. H. S. (2011). Why health care process performance measures can have different relationships to outcomes for patients and hospitals: Understanding the ecological fallacy. *American Journal of Public Health, 101*, 1635–1642. https://doi.org/10.2105/AJPH.2011.300153

Fonarow, G. C., Abraham, W. T., Albert, N. M., Stough, W. G., Gheorghiade, M., Greenberg, B. H., O'Connor, C. M., Pieper, K., Sun, J. L., & Young, J. B. (2007). Association between performance measures and clinical outcomes for patients hospitalized with heart failure. *Journal of the American Medical Association, 297*, 61–70.

Forsey, L. M., & O'Rourke, M. W. (2013, July 22–26). *Optimizing hospital RN role competency leads to improved patient outcomes.* Presentation at Sigma Theta Tau 24th International Nursing Research Congress, Prague, Czech Republic.

Fromm, E. (1956). *The art of loving.* Harper & Row.

Gale, E. A. M. (2004). The Hawthorne studies—A fable for our times? *QJM: An International Journal of Medicine, 97*, 439–449. https://doi.org/10.1093/qjmed/hch070

Graetz, F. (2002). Strategic thinking versus strategic planning: Towards understanding the complementarities. *Management Decision, 40*, 456–462.

Graham, M. (2012, March 9). Big data and the end of theory? *The Guardian.* https://www .theguardian.com/news/datablog/2012/mar/09/big-data-theory

Haddon, R. M. (1989, May/June). The final frontier: Nursing in the emerging healthcare environment. *Nursing Economic$, 7,* 151.

Haines, S. G. (1998). *The manager's pocket guide to systems thinking & learning.* HRD Press: Amhurst Massachusetts.

Hibbard, J., & Greene, J. (2013). What the evidence shows about patient activation: Better health outcomes and care experiences; fewer data on costs. *Health Affairs, 32*(2). http://dx .doi.org/https://doi.org/10.1377/hlthaff.2012.1061

Hilbert, M., & López, P. (2011, April 1). The world's technological capacity to store, communicate, and compute information. *Science, 332*, 60–65.

Hussain, S. T., Lei, S., Akram, T., Haider, M. J., Hussain, S. H., & Ali, M. (2018). Kurt Lewin's change model: A critical review of the role of leadership and employee involvement in organizational change. *Journal of Innovation & Knowledge, 3*(3), 123–127.

Institute for Health Improvement. (2023a). About us. https://www.ihi.org/about/Pages /History.aspx

Institute for Health Improvement. (2023b). What is the triple aim? https://www.ihi.org /Topics/TripleAim/Pages/Overview.aspx#:~:text=It%20is%20IHI's%20belief%20 that,capita%20cost%20of%20health%20care

Institute for Health Metrics and Evaluation (IHME). (2020). *Financing global health 2020: The impact of COVID-19.* IHME.

Institute of Medicine. (2001, March 1). *Crossing the quality chasm: A new health system for the 21st century.* National Academy Press.

Interaction Design Foundation. (2020). 5 stages in the design thinking process. https://www.interaction-design.org/literature/article/5-stages-in-the-design-thinking-process

International Business Machines. (2023). *Big Data: Overview* [Fact sheet]. https://www.ibm.com/analytics/big-data-analytics#:~:text=What%20is%20big%20data%20exactly,high%20velocity%20and%20high%20variety

Interprofessional Education Collaborative Expert Panel. (2011). *Core competencies for interprofessional collaborative practice: Report of an expert panel.* Interprofessional Education Collaborative.

Kagan, O., Littlejohn, J., Nadel, H., & Leary, M. (2021, September 30). Evolution of nurse-led hackathons, incubators, and accelerators from an innovation ecosystem perspective. *The Online Journal of Issues in Nursing, 26*(3). https://doi.org/10.3912/OJIN.Vol26No03Man03

Kalil, T. (2012, March 29). *Big data is a big deal* [Blog post]. https://obamawhitehouse.archives.gov/blog/2012/03/29/big-data-big-deal

Kanter, R. M. (1996). When a thousand flowers bloom: Structural, collective, and social conditions for innovation in organizations. In P. S. Myers (Ed.), *Knowledge management and organizational design* (pp. 93–131). Routledge. doi.org/10.1016/B978-0-7506-9749-1.50010-7

Ketokivi, M., Bromiley, P., & Awaysheh, A. (2021). Making theoretically informed choices in specifying panel-data models. *Production and Operations Management, 30*(7), 2069–2076.

Kirzinger, A., Montero, A., Hamel, L., & Brodie, M. (2022, April 14). 5 charts about public opinion on the Affordable Care Act. *KFF.*

Klein, K. J., & Kozlowski, S. W. J. (2000). *Multilevel theory, research, and methods in organizations: Foundations, extensions, and new directions.* Jossey-Bass.

Kohn, L.T., Corrigan, J. M., & Donaldson, M. S. (Eds.). (2000). *To err is human: Building a safer health system.* Institute of Medicine (US) Committee on Quality of Health Care in America. National Academy Press.

Kouzes, J. M., & Posner, B. Z. (2000). *Leadership practices inventory: Psychometric properties.* John Wiley & Sons.

Kritsonis, A. (2005). Comparison of change theories. *International Journal of Scholarly Academic Intellectual Diversity, 8*(1), 1–7.

Liedtka, J. (1998). Linking strategic thinking with strategic planning. *Strategy and Leadership, 26*, 30–35.

Lippitt, R., Watson, J., & Westley, B. (1958). *The dynamics of planned change.* Harcourt, Brace & World.

Liu, W., Edwards, H., & Courtney, M. (2009). Review of continuing professional education in case management for nurses. *Nurse Education Today, 29*(5), 488–492.

Loos, N., & O'Rourke, M. W. (2012, November). *Autonomy, job satisfaction and quality of care: Barriers and facilitators of a role based approach to practice within the context of the essentials of magnetism* [Conference paper]. Sigma Theta Tau International Conference, Brisbane, Australia.

Makary, M. A., & Daniel, M. (2016). Medical error—the third leading cause of death in the US. *BMJ*, *353*(2139). doi:10.1136/bmj.i2139

Mandelbrot, B. B. (2008). How fractals can explain what's wrong with Wall Street. *Scientific American*, *15*(9). https://www.scientificamerican.com/article/multifractals-explain-wall -street/

Mensik, J. (2013, January). *The nurse manager's guide to innovative and effective staffing*. Sigma Theta Tau International.

Mercado, S. E. (2020). NAHQ's perspective on healthcare quality as business strategy. *The Journal for Healthcare Quality (JHQ)*, *42*(2), 65.

Merriam-Webster. (n.d.). *Science definition & meaning*. Merriam-Webster. https://www .merriam-webster.com/dictionary/science

Merton, R. K. (1936, December). The unanticipated consequences of purposive social action. *American Sociological Review*, *1*, 894–904.

Mevawala, A. S., Strunk, F. A., Haghiri-Vijeh, R., Corless, I. B., Ramaswamy, P., Kamp, K. J., Scott, S., & Gray, S. (2021). Scientific global nursing hackathon experience. *Nurse Educator*, *46*(6), E154–E157. https://doi.org/10.1097/NNE.0000000000001066

Miller, J. G. (1978). *Living systems*. McGraw-Hill.

Mostafazadeh-Bora, M. (2020). The Hawthorne effect in observational studies: Threat or opportunity? *Infection Control & Hospital Epidemiology*, *41*(4), 491–491.

Mostashari, F. (2014). Farzad Mostashari, MD, answers why data is "oxygen" for innovation [Interview by AJMCTV.com]. https://www.ajmc.com/view/farzad-mostashari-md-answers -why-data-is-oxygen-for-innovation

Murray, E. (2017). *Nursing leadership and management: for patient safety and quality care*. FA Davis.

National Academy of Medicine. (2023). About us. https://nam.edu/about-the-nam/

National Academies of Sciences, Engineering, and Medicine. (2021). *The future of nursing 2020–2030: Charting a path to achieve health equity*. The National Academies Press. https://doi.org/10.17226/25982

National Quality Forum. (2023a). What we do. https://www.qualityforum.org/what_we_do .aspx

National Quality Forum. (2023b). NQF's history. https://www.qualityforum.org/about_nqf /history/

National Research Council. (2011). *The future of nursing: Leading change, advancing health*. The National Academies Press.

National Science Foundation (NSF). (2021, June). Elementary and secondary public school expenditure in the United States as a percentage of GDP in 2018, by state. U.S. public school expenditure by state as a percentage of GDP. *Statista*.

Nelson, E. C., Batalden, P. B., & Godfrey, M. M. (2007). *Quality by design: A clinical microsystems approach*. Jossey-Bass.

Nelson, J. (2022). *Economic effects of five illustrative single-payer health care systems.* Working Paper 2022-02 (No. 57637).

Newhouse, J. P. (1992). Medical care costs: How much welfare loss? *Journal of Economic Perspectives, 6,* 3–23.

Nundy, S., Cooper, L. A., & Mate, K. S. (2022). The quintuple aim for health care improvement: A new imperative to advance health equity. *Journal of the American Medical Association, 327*(6), 521–522. https://doi.org/10.1001/jama.2021.25181

Patient-Centered Outcomes Research Institute. (2023). About us. https://www.pcori.org/about/about-pcori

Piantadosi, S. (1994). Invited commentary: Ecologic biases. *American Journal Epidemiology, 139,* 761–764.

Prochaska, J. O., & DiClemente, C. C. (1984). *The transtheoretical approach: Towards a systematic eclectic framework.* Dow Jones Irwin.

Prokesch, S. (2009, January 1). How GE teaches teams to lead change. *Harvard Business Review,* pp. 1–9. https://hbr.org/2009/01/how-ge-teaches-teams-to-lead-change

Quisenberry, E. (2021). How does standard work lead to better patient safety? https://www.virginiamasoninstitute.org/how-does-standard-work-lead-to-better-patient-safety/

Robert Wood Johnson Foundation. (2011). *Health policy snapshot: Workforce* [Issue brief]. http://www.rwjf.org/content/dam/farm/reports/issue_briefs/2011/rwjf72058

Robinson, W. S. (1950). Ecological correlations and the behavior of individuals. *American Sociological Review, 15,* 351–357.

Rogers, E. M. (2003). *Diffusion of innovations* (5th ed.). Free Press.

Rundio, A. (2016). *The nurse manager's guide to budgeting & finance* (2nd ed.). Sigma Theta Tau International.

Safar, J., Defields, C., Fulop, A., Dowd, M., & Zavod, M. (2007, February 17). Meeting business goals and managing office bandwidth: A predictive model for organizational change. *Journal of Change Management, 6,* 87–98.

Scott, K. A., & Mensik, J. S. (2010). Creating the conditions for breakthrough clinical performance. *Nurse Leader, 8,* 48–52. https://doi.org/10.1016/j.mnl.2010.05.004

Shortell, S. M., & Schmittdiel, J. (2004). Prepaid groups and organized delivery systems: Promise, performance, and potential. In A. C. Enthoven, & L. A. Tollen (Eds.), *Toward a twenty-first century health system: The contributions and promise of prepaid group practice* (pp. W5-420–W5-433). Jossey-Bass.

Shrank, W. H., Rogstad, T. L., & Parekh, N. (2019). Waste in the US health care system: Estimated costs and potential for savings. *Journal of the American Medical Association, 322*(15), 1501–1509. https://doi.org/10.1001/jama.2019.13978

Simon, H. (1957). *Models of man, social and rational: Mathematical essays on rational human behavior in a social setting* (pp. 196–279). John Wiley & Sons.

Sinnott, M., Mullins, J. M., & Simmons, K. L. (2020). How do you implement value-based care methodologies in dentistry with existing dental organizational paradigms? *Journal of Public Health Dentistry, 80,* S104–S108.

References

Sivers, D. (2010, February). How to start a movement [Video file]. https://www.ted.com
/talks/derek_sivers_how_to_start_a_movement

Six Sigma Institute. (n.d.). Six Sigma DMAIC Process—Define Phase—Change Acceleration
Process (CAP). https://www.sixsigma-institute.org/Six_Sigma_DMAIC_Process_Define
_Phase_Change_Acceleration_Process_CAP.php

Smith, M. A. (2011). Are you a transformational leader? *Nursing Management, 42*, 44–50.
https://doi.org/10.1097/01.NUMA.0000403279.04379.6a

State Health Agency. (n.d.). Retrieved from http://en.wikipedia.org/wiki/State_health_agency

Statista. (2022, December). *U.S. national health expenditure as percent of GDP from 1960 to
2020*. https://www.statista.com/statistics/184968/us-health-expenditure-as-percent-of-gdp
-since-1960/

Stephens, M. (2010, December 15). *7 reasons why you need to work for a big company* [Blog
post]. http://onstartups.com/tabid/3339/bid/33111/7-Reasons-Why-You-Need-To-Work-For
-A-Big-Company.aspx

Swensen, S. J., Meyer, G. S., Nelson, E. C., Hunt, G. C., Jr., Pryor, D. B., Weissberg, J. I., Kaplan,
G. S., Daley, J., Yates, G. R., Chassin, M. R., James, B. C., & Berwick, D. M. (2010, January 20).
Cottage industry to postindustrial care—The revolution in health care delivery. *New England
Journal of Medicine, 362*, 772–774. https://doi.org/10.1056/NEJMp0911199

Szczerba, R. J., & Huesch, M. D. (2012, September 10). Why technology matters as much as
science in improving healthcare. *BMC Medical Informatics and Decision Making, 12*, 103.

Taylor, F. W. (1911). *The principles of scientific management*. Harper Brothers.

Technology. (n.d.). http://en.wikipedia.org/wiki/Technology

Virkstis, K. (2014). What is top of license nursing practice? https://www.advisory.com/topics
/nursing/2013/04/achieving-top-of-license-nursing-practice

Voelpel, S., Leibold, M., & Tekie, E. (2004). The wheel of business model reinvention: How to
reshape your business model to leapfrog competitors. *Journal of Change Management, 4*,
259–276.

Von Der Linn, B. (2009). Overview of GE's Change Acceleration Process (CAP). Agility science:
Bob Von Der Linn's Change Management and Human Performance Technology Blog. https://
bvonderlinn.wordpress.com/2009/01/25/overview-of-ges-change-acceleration-process-cap/

Wasson, J. H. (2019). Insights from organized crime for disorganized health care. *The Journal
of Ambulatory Care Management, 42*(2), 138.

Watkins, M. (2007, April 20). *How to think strategically* [Blog post]. https://hbr.org/2007/04
/how-to-think-strategically-1

Weber, M. (1968). *Economy and society: An outline of interpretive sociology.* (pp. 956–1005).
University of California Press.

Werner, R. M., & Bradlow, E. T. (2006). Relationship between Medicare's hospital compare
performance measures and mortality rates. *Journal of the American Medical Association,
296*, 2694–2702. https://doi.org/10.1001/jama.296.22.2694

Westley, F., Zimmerman, B., & Patton, M. (2007). *Getting to maybe.* Vintage Canada.

Wheatley, M. J. (2006). *Leadership and the new science: Discovering order in a chaotic world* (3rd ed.). Berrett-Koehler.

White House, Department of Defense. (2014). The budget for fiscal year 2014. https://www.govinfo.gov/app/collection/BUDGET/2014

Winer, M., & Ray, K. (1994). *Collaboration handbook: Creating, sustaining, and enjoying the journey.* Amherst H. Wilder Foundation.

Wong, C. A., Cummings, G. G., & Ducharme, D. (2013). The relationship between nursing leadership and patient outcomes: A systematic review update. *Journal of Nursing Management, 21,* 709–724.

World Health Organization. (2005). What is a health system? https://cdn.who.int/media/docs/default-source/documents/health-systems-strengthening-glossary.pdf

World Health Organization. (2010). Key components of a well functioning healthcare system [Pamphlet]. /https://apps.who.int/iris/bitstream/handle/10665/258734/9789241564052-eng.pdf

World Health Organization. (2023a). About WHO. https://www.who.int/about

World Health Organization. (2023b). The Triple Billion targets: A visual summary of methods to deliver impact. https://www.who.int/data/stories/the-triple-billion-targets-a-visual-summary-of-methods-to-deliver-impact

Index

D

E

I

J

K

L

Q

R

S

T

About the Author

Jennifer S. Mensik Kennedy, PhD, MBA, RN, NEA-BC, FAAN, is currently an assistant professor at the Oregon Health and Science University School of Nursing in Portland Oregon and president of the American Nurses Association. Mensik Kennedy is a sought-after presenter and prolific author. Her books include *The Nurse Managers Guide to Innovative Staffing 2ⁿᵈ ed.* She co-authored *Lead Like a Nurse, A Nurse's Step-By-Step Guide to Transitioning to the Professional Nurse Role,* and *The Power of Ten, 2ⁿᵈ ed.* and contributed a chapter to the book *The Career Handoff: A Healthcare Leader's Guide to Knowledge & Wisdom Transfer across Generations.*

Mensik Kennedy has held numerous high-profile leadership positions within the nursing profession. She served as president of the Arizona Nurses Association from 2007–2010. Nationally, Mensik Kennedy has served as treasurer, second vice president, and director-at-large on the American Nurses Association board of directors. Additionally, she held the role of governor of nursing practice for the Western Institute of Nursing from 2010–2014.

Mensik Kennedy earned a PhD from the University of Arizona College of Nursing with a focus on health systems and a minor in public administration from the Eller College of Management. Mensik Kennedy's MBA degree is from the University of Phoenix, while her BSN degree is from Washington State University. She also holds an ADN degree from Wenatchee Valley College-North. Mensik Kennedy was inducted as a fellow to the American Academy of Nursing in 2014.